The ABC's Of Mental Health:

Ten Chapters To Healing

Dr. Noel Goldberg, Psy.D

The ABC's Of Mental Health:
Ten Chapters To Healing

DEDICATION

This book is dedicated to all of the Veterans from the United States of America, who have taught me and allowed me to teach them how to cope with mental difficulties. This book is also dedicated to all of the struggling individuals out there looking for answers to life's circumscribed set of problems.

ACKNOWLEDGEMENTS

We set off on the course of life to make some type of memorable contribution to our world in the hopes of improving it or leaving it better than when we entered it. We do not know what that mark will be, but we desire to leave such a mark. Whether or not I will ever leave such a mark, my hope is that this book finds its way into people's hands to enrich their lives and improve their lot in life. That is my goal. I am not sure if it's such a grand contribution and who knows, maybe I will be able to contribute more, but I am hoping that this will be my lasting mark. And upon this mark, I would like to thank all of the people who have assisted me in not only writing this book, but who have inspired me to develop the material I wrote about. This includes all of the professionals who have trained me in my life at the University of Massachusetts at Amherst, State University of New York at Albany, the University of North Carolina at Chapel Hill, Duke University, the College of William and Mary, Old Dominion University, Eastern Virginia Medical School, and Norfolk State University. I also would like to thank the staff at the Albany Consortium and Virginia Consortium, as well as the Veteran Affairs Medical Centers at which I have trained and worked.

I also gratefully acknowledge the time at the Washington, DC Veteran Affairs Medical Center (VAMC), without which the practicing of this model would never have been attempted nor completed. It was through my work with veterans that I was able to design, implement, and improve this model.

Closer to home, I would like to thank my wife Malki, my son Ashlon, my parents and sister, and my friends for their continued support throughout all of graduate school and my career. Additionally, I would like to thank all of the faculty along the way who have helped me during my pursuit of a higher education.

Special thanks also goes to Dr. John Thibodeau for providing continued support throughout my career, and Dr. Sam Levinson for his wise advisement and career counseling. In particular, I would like to recognize the following individuals for their unique contribution to this book: Matt Cail for the cover page; my editor, Martin J. Coffee; and my director of marketing.

And to all of the individuals who made this model a reality, thank you. With all my heart I hope you can use this model in your daily life to improve your life.

CONTENTS

I. INTRODUCTION

I have been working and training in psychology for the past 20 years and continue to try to better understand not only the world around me, but people's behavior. While integrating this vast amount of learned knowledge and experience, I began to develop a philosophy or way to view mental illness that I thought would be helpful to others. This viewpoint translated my knowledge and experience of mental illness into basic concepts that the layperson can readily learn and apply.

It has transcended into a teaching tool, whereby others might benefit from my integration of a variety of mental health issues and readily applicable solutions. This teaching tool or model began to help many individuals, especially the Military Veterans under my care. To this end, I have begun to transcribe these integrated concepts in the hopes that others can benefit from my written "teachings."

I hereby present my model entitled "The ABC's of Mental Health." If learned and applied to everyday life, I think many individuals can learn to better control their lives, and more importantly, their reactions to life.

The BASICS

My model is simple. The first concept implements a triangle as an aid to understanding it. It is what drives all mental activity.

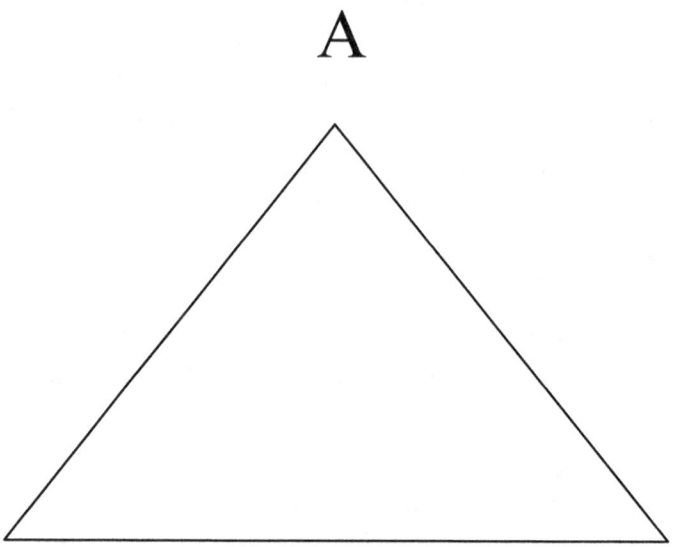

This triangle is comprised of three areas that encompass all mental issues. These are Affect, Behavior and Cognitions or simply put the ABC's. All of our mental processes entail Affect or our feelings or emotions, our Behavior, and our Cognitions or thoughts. Some people like to use the acronym (B.E.T. symbolizing Behavior, Emotions, and Thoughts), but I prefer referring to it as the ABC model as it implies simplicity.

This model can be used to guide mental health because there are various areas where one can intervene to change outcomes. Specifically, if one is depressed, you can work on changing your behavior or your thoughts. Behavioral changes can include exercise, diet, employment, relationships, repetitive patterns, rewards, and various other behavioral difficulties.

Our depressive cognitions or thoughts might be "I am no good" or "I will always fail" or "I will never be loved." These thoughts need to be changed into "I am a good person" or "I will succeed" or "I am deserving of love." Sometimes these negative thoughts are deeply engrained by family and life experience, and although they may be difficult to change, one can consistently work to change them. If the application of this model doesn't lead to lasting change, professional help may then be required. Other lifestyle changes that can lead to better mental health include a solid structure, improved communication, new coping strategies, or adhering to medication usage.

Most people perform better with greater structure, especially on a daily basis. In inpatient hospital units and in some outpatient treatment centers, a very strong structure helps patients adjust. In everyday life, our structure includes our sleep, eating, exercise, and putting time into pleasurable activities. If we create an individualized, manageable structure, then we can readily identify where our difficulties come from. Let me elaborate.

Example 1. Let's say you go to bed at 11PM, awake at 7AM, go to the bathroom, brush your teeth, eat breakfast, shower, make your bed, get dressed, and leave for work by 8AM. Later, you have lunch at 1PM and return home at 6PM. This is your daily structure over which you have some control, even if you can't change your work hours because you still have a structure to your life. Extending this structure or schedule, you may go to the gym in the morning or during mid-

3

evening, prepare dinner until 7:30PM, watch TV while eating, start to relax at 9PM and by 11PM, get ready for bedtime. This very structured or scheduled lifestyle might have some strong benefits if you are prone to mood swings or anxiety. Specifically, everything has been predictable (bedtime, meal time…) so that if you begin to decompensate (or not feel psychologically strong) you can determine the cause (i.e., not getting enough sleep, eating poorly…).

I thoroughly believe there is a cause to our problems, whether purely environment or physical (for those with chemical imbalances). For example, let's say you're a married man and keep to the above schedule. However, you don't enjoy your job and instead of going to the gym, you decide to take a break and after work go with some buddies to drink. You seem to enjoy this activity and expand it to three times a week and on Sunday you watch football while drinking beer. Unfortunately, on Sunday you drink too much, have trouble sleeping and call in sick Monday. The next week, it's the same problem except that you show up to work but are unable to function at the level you usually do because you were up late partying and didn't get enough sleep. Thus a new pattern has begun. Because you are "hung over," you are increasingly short-tempered at work and at home. Fights ensue in both places. It creates difficulties in your marriage and at work, with you eventually getting fired. Now you begin to really feel depressed for good reasons. The tension has increased at home, especially with being unemployed, as you spend more time with your spouse and money gets tight.

As illustrated by this example, you changed your structure, began to cope inappropriately by drinking alcohol excessively, and through both environmental causes of loss of job and fighting with your wife, you find yourself depressed. If you continue on this path, we can identify two problems: first alcohol and eventually clinical depression. Simplifying the life equation, there is certainly a well-defined cause-effect relationship occurring here. However, there are many places to intervene by creating a solid structure, such as going to the gym instead of the bar, so prevention could have begun early.

The trajectory of a depressive cycle can be improved or worsened in multiple places by multiple pathways or points. In the above example, intervention can occur by 1) maintaining your self-created schedule or structure; 2) abstaining from alcohol; 3) beginning antidepressants; 4) improving your communication; and 5) finding more appropriate coping mechanisms. These areas will be discussed in greater detail in the subsequent chapters.

Example 2: You're a single woman working 9-5 and have a strong support system. Let's say you have been dating a guy for five years and he suddenly tells you that he is not interested in having a family. You are saddened by his decision and by the amount of time you have invested in this relationship. Thus you begin to feel "blue." Because you are also having problems at your boring job, the depression becomes worse. Sound familiar? However, you sense you're feeling depressed and friends suggest a particular herbal product on the market that might help. You begin trying St. John's Wart to deal with your feelings of depression and its starts to work... somewhat. Things are starting to improve, right? Wrong!

Hypothetically, let's say that you have trouble breaking off this relationship because you love this man, and let's extend the reasoning by saying that you have some low self-esteem, being that you're 30 years old and doubt another man will want you. You question what you have to offer someone new, which leads you to thinking you should be thankful you have such a "wonderful" man in your life. This reasoning seems logical. Right? You continue in your relationship because you're afraid to leave and continue having sex with your boyfriend. You also stay in your job because of financial circumstances and you are not motivated enough to apply to other jobs. Now, we have a few ways to go.

Because of depression, you might seek to escape from your current relationship or your boyfriend might want a break because of your constant low motivation and mood. If infidelity occurs, each partner can complicate matters by bringing the possibility of sexually transmitted diseases into the relationship. You are also aware that if you're not happy, typically neither is your partner. If infidelity does not occur, there is the possibility that one of the members in the relationship will begin to drink, use illegal drugs, or act out in other ways. Although this happens more times than not, let's stay with our present example of "maintaining" the current relationship strictly with the above mentioned psychological issues of dissimilar future goals, unsatisfactory employment, and increasing depression alleviated somewhat by St. John's Wart. Thus, you continue in this relationship and become more concerned when you miss your monthly period. A self-administered pregnancy test brings a positive result. You're pregnant! This is confirmed with a visit to your Primary Care Physician.

Perhaps you think this is not realistic, right? Wrong! A little known fact backed by medical research has shown that when a woman takes St. John's Wart in conjunction with birth control pills, the St. John's Wart can counteract the effects of the "pill." Most women don't know that. Thus if you really weren't depressed before, you will be depressed now because you have an unwanted pregnancy.

Let's review the circumstances of this example again. You're relationship has no future, you have a man who does not want a family, a job you don't enjoy, self-esteem issues abound, and all this most definitely will lead to depression. You can plot how the rest turns out.

In this scenario, there are various places to intervene, from addressing the relationship by communicating, changing jobs, addressing self-esteem through psychotherapy, building successes, or expressing your feelings, and/or taking appropriate medications. The suggested course in the latter situation is antidepressants that are regulated by the Food and Drug Administration (FDA) versus herbal supplements that are not standardized or regulated.

You can help yourself CHANGE to prevent increased problems of depression and anxiety by identifying the problems early. Just like in medicine, if you catch a disease early, you have a better chance of preventing it from becoming worse. Intervening early with mental problems can have the same result as long as it is addressed early before it becomes a problematic pattern.

To understand what impedes our mental health and our management of it, we need to recognize the elements of the model. The expounded graphic displayed on the following page highlights the interaction or bidirectionality of the three cornerstones of mental health: AFFECT, BEHAVIOR, AND COGNITIONS. From the following triangle, those three central cornerstones of this model are displayed. How they work separately and together is the key to understanding and preventing psychological problems.

AFFECT

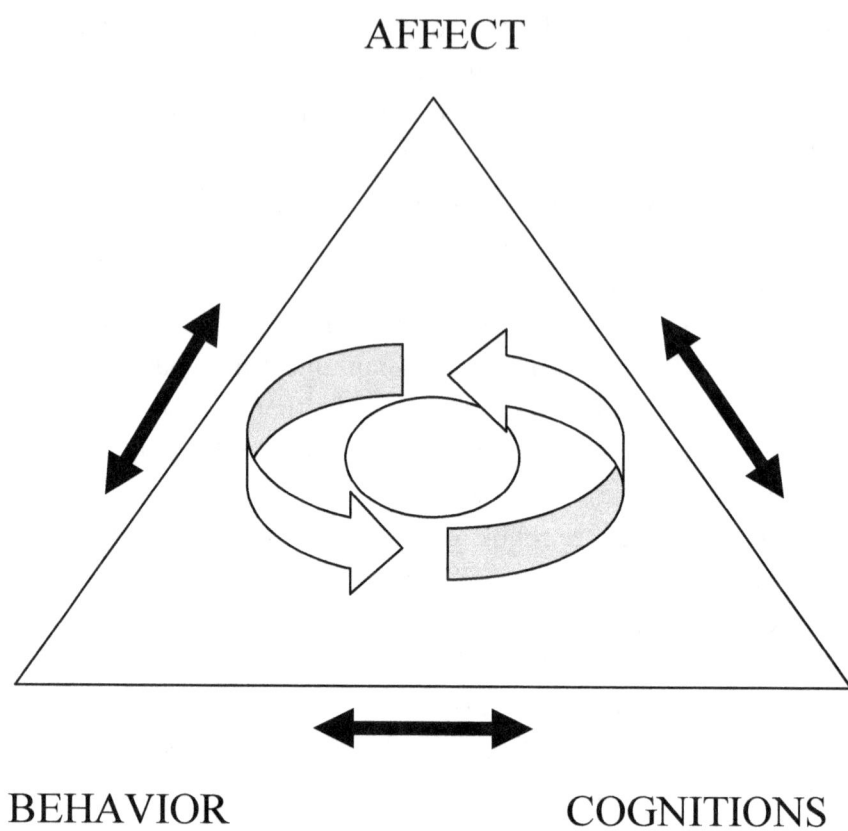

BEHAVIOR   COGNITIONS

The arrows signify bidirectionality, meaning that each corner or area can influence the other in multiple ways: affect can influence behavior or cognitions, behavior can influence affect or cognitions, cognitions can influence behavior or affect.

II. AFFECT

Affect (feelings or emotions) is a very important part of daily life and typically an important area to focus on when undergoing psychotherapy. People generally try not to feel and avoid such feelings or emotions. As a result, they can be quite delayed in allowing themselves to feel, which can negatively affect relationships.

In psychotherapy, a large focus of treatment is to enable patients to begin to identify their feelings and begin to actually process these feelings. By process, I mean to fully "feel" their emotions. For example, when one talks about the death of a parent, someone they deeply cared about, they can feel sad and experience the sadness. A real testament to this feeling would be to cry, maybe not uncontrollably but to really experience the sadness through tears. In this way, the individual is allowing themself to feel and process this emotion. Some call this a catharsis or release of emotional energy, but I call it making the feeling or emotion *real*. By doing this, you are validating your experience and feeling. You are in the act of experiencing sadness versus saying "I am sad," a statement that seems devoid of the emotional impact.

Some people prefer to go through life without "feeling" the emotion while others experience the emotion, but do not fully "feel" the emotion. Is this okay? Well, affect is a central part of our life and without feeling it, you miss out on much of what life has to offer. There are reasons for your behavior because, psychologically speaking, there were events in your life where, in order to survive, you had to close off your feelings. The problem with using this type of coping skill now as an adult, as

9

opposed to when you were younger or a child, is that it limits the fullness of your life. More specifically, it prevents you from interacting on all the levels possible, like a six cylinder engine that is firing on only four cylinders. Since you are not "running on all cylinders," this functioning puts you at a distinct disadvantage in life.

Veteran patients of mine have asked, "Why do we need to feel? I have survived without feeling all my life." In exploring this question and the Veteran's life experience, we discover that the Veteran, in order to cope with the difficulties of life, shut out their feelings. For example, in a combat situation, a properly trained soldier would not survive if they became overwrought with emotions during battle. It was normal to witness a buddy getting injured or killed. Soldiers are trained to move on and survive. They do not process the fear, sadness, hurt, and anger or the multitude of other emotions that might be stirred up and bottled up.

This lack of processing actually begins early in life because children have also learned to adapt this coping mechanism for survival's sake. If a child is raised in a chaotic and violent household, they learn not to deal with their feelings in order to survive. This adaptation or coping is very important to the CHILD in their specific life circumstances (i.e., raised with alcoholic or abusive parents). Unfortunately, as adults, we continue to avoid dealing with, addressing, or processing one's feelings and this has the distinct disadvantage of making life more black and white instead of gray. It limits our ability to fully "feel" or live life with all of the wonderful emotions available to experience.

The movie *Pleasantville* provides a colorful example to elaborate. In *Pleasantville*, the characters went through life without being able to see color. Color symbolizes emotion, both good and bad, and when you go through life without emotion, you miss out on a great many things. Just as you are unable to experience euphoria, pleasure, happiness, and bliss, you also try to avoid pain, anger, hurt, disappointment, sadness, misery, and loneliness. By not opening yourself up to your feelings, you minimize your life. Unfortunately, there is always a cost to coping this way and the cost is missing out on the positives of life, the fullness of life, and the inherent depth in relationships. Without rain, plants do not grow and they die. With rain, plants thrive. Without sadness, we do not appreciate happiness nor do we feel fully. Experiencing sadness and happiness brings out the true realism of life's feelings.

CONTINUUM OF FEELINGS

Within the ABC Model of Mental Health, I would like to discuss the continuum of feelings, which includes extremes. What are extremes? Extremes are excessive responses or feelings that typically include two parts, the quantity aspect and the quality aspect. Typically, people who have continuous extreme feelings in their daily lives are unable to modulate their feelings and have many problems interacting with others. They seem to overreact and probably are labeled emotional, over-emotional, unstable, passionate, "intense," excessive, full of drama or crazy.

When a person is open to feelings, they are able to experience the full spectrum of feelings, between like and love, attraction and lust, or annoyance and hate. The full spectrum includes the endpoints as well as all the points in the middle. These previous examples are the extremes on the continuum of the quality of feelings. While it is perfectly fine to experience intense or extreme feelings, it becomes another story when intense feelings pervade your daily life.

When I talk about emotional extremes, I refer to people who always have these extreme feelings, like having trouble with anger management and always feeling like they are in a rage. Or, people feel quite the opposite, completely lacking any feelings of anger. These are both extremes in the quality of your response and, in some respect, the quantity.

As an example, if someone slights you in your daily interactions and you become full of intense anger, this is probably an over-reaction. From this over-reaction, your heart rate increases, blood pressure goes up, you might begin to sweat, and your breathing increases. All of this from your reaction to a slight perceived as personal. Multiply this reaction by the hundreds of slights you receive in a week and one easily begins to see how unhealthy this approach to daily interactions can be.

My argument is that a continuous, extreme response is unhealthy and can be controlled. You can learn how to modulate your reactions by using the ABC approach. Let's say while driving to or from work, another driver cuts you off on the road and you begin to get very angry. You never know when this anger can cause major problems, from physical damage like a brain aneurism, stroke, or heart attack to a car accident by following them, tailgating, ramming into their rear end or losing control of your vehicle. Not convinced? Let's go with a specific example that happened in the late 1990's in Long Island, NY. A male driver was going home on the Southern State Expressway—commonly referred to as the world's longest parking lot because of traffic jams—driving along, probably annoyed at something from work when another driver was weaving in and out of traffic, obviously in a hurry and extremely frustrated with the pace of travel. He continued going in and out of traffic and cut this man off, who was still irritated from his job. Initially he cursed the other driver out, but that wasn't enough. He then began to follow him, driving erratically and tailgating, but our man wasn't satisfied with this plan of action, so he decided to summon the man to pull over, continuing to shout expletives in the process. As they both pulled over on the shoulder of the busy highway, our angry man got out of his car, opened up his trunk, pulled out his hunting crossbow, loaded it, and as the other driver got out of his vehicle and walked toward the man, the crossbow was fired and the arrow pierced the man's heart. Don't believe it? It's a true story, as reported in the *Long Island Newsday*.

What is so important about this example? The man was unable to control his anger response and it cost him dearly. In all probability, this man was not so angry with the other driver, but rather a combination of events or past history that led him to the point of no return. Regardless of his past circumstances, the fact is that he had an excessive overreaction to what normal people would simply consider poor or non-courteous driving. Because of his aggressive behavior and his inability to deal with his anger and rage, this man is now serving a life sentence for killing the other driver and his behavior has also affected his family since they no longer have their father/husband to support them and raise them.

What can be learned from this example? It is the ability to learn how to control your reactions, feelings, and limit displays of extreme behavior or feelings. You can control your reaction and learn to modulate the reaction by using the biggest muscle you have, your brain.

Daniel Goleman, the author of the bestselling book *Emotional Intelligence*, defined a term he called "emotional hijacking," where an individual loses the ability to think clearly once he hits this "zone." It's similar to the red line on a car engine, where it is very risky to drive in this area or zone, unless you wish to blow up the engine. Mr. Goleman talked about the process of emotional hijacking and how thousands of years ago it served homosapiens well by allowing them to avoid danger when dinosaurs or other large creatures were around. To save your life, you needed to react quickly and wisely in terms of flight or fight. He also talked about how our internal, inherited emotional circuitry has not changed and kept pace with the advances of modern day technology. This process of emotional hijacking is usually found with our extreme reactions and feelings. Whether it is intense anger or rage, despair, catatonic depression or manic energy, an extreme feeling or reaction repeated can be very unhealthy.

You can begin to manage your reactions and feelings by gaining insight into how you process an event or stimuli, and identify your reaction. By understanding how you react and knowing that your options include changing or intervening within affect, behavior, or cognitions, you can begin to develop alternative ways to react. Let's remember from the ABC's that you have 3 pathways to intervene and change your response. Remember...the extremes on the affective or feelings continuum point to the importance of finding a middle ground in life.

What is also important in emotional reactions is the quantity or amount of feeling a person experiences. If a person is continually flooded with excessive feelings, then this extreme can also cause major concerns. Picture a woman who cannot

14

control herself and is constantly crying. Ever been around a person who was so emotional that you didn't know how to respond? They can be exhausting, always filled with emotion in all aspects of their lives.

In Yiddish, they have a great term for this called "chazarim," which basically means chaos. These folks generate an atmosphere or aura of chaos as they fill other people around them with intense emotionality. It almost feels like the Tasmanian Devil approaching, turning things upside down and leaving a path of destruction in its wake. People like this go beyond reacting with extreme emotions because there is never an escape from this extreme emotionality. In every interaction, they are always over-emotional. Sometimes they are labeled "sensitive" if they are prone to crying; if they are prone to confrontation and fighting, they are just plain "assertive/aggressive." This type of behavior, always experiencing extreme emotion, is unhealthy physically and negatively affects your interactions with others (especially when people try to avoid you).

CONTRAST

It's funny, but I also like to look at the contrast of feelings, like love versus hate or sadness against happiness. Let me extend my train of thought. Within the extremes on the continuum, a very powerful notion usually expressed by behaviorists is that you cannot simultaneously feel two distinctly opposite feelings, like feeling depressed while feeling happy or laughing at the same time. These are called incompatible responses or behaviors. For example, you can't do well in school while you're getting in trouble. These behaviors are incongruent. It's similar to the opposites of life and death, depression and mania, and mental health versus mental illness.

Why is understanding the concept of contrasts or polar opposites so important? This dictum, that of the contrasts of life, highlights an important principle of mental health, that of incongruent states. Within this concept, you can intervene and be guided by polar opposite feeling states.

While extremes in behavior are not the goal, knowing the direct opposite of a feeling state, like the extreme of sadness as happiness, can help you attain an alternative feeling state to the one you are currently experiencing. You can recognize your current state and move out of it by working to obtain the exact opposite state, even if the exact opposite state on the continuum is not achieved. Remember, the continuum exists on a scale (like 0 to 100) and by moving off the extreme low number (say 0 to say 25), you at least raise yourself out of the current low feeling state. By recognizing your low feeling state and knowing that you must move toward your alternate goal, you have a better chance to achieve that goal even if it is initially not the optimum state.

For example, if you recognize that you are sad, you can try for a feeling state of happiness. If the number zero were assigned to your sadness, meaning extreme sadness or despair, your immediate goal would be to move away from that extreme negative feeling. Then hopefully you can work up to extreme cheerfulness or euphoria.

Applying the ABC's, you can work towards this positive state by intervening in any of the three ABC areas of affect, behavior or cognition. Typically, the easiest way to change this state (although it does not feel easy) is to change your behavior. If you're sad, you have a choice. You can either validate your sadness—as if your favorite pet died, and help process that feeling by looking over old photos or videos of your pet and simply grieve—or you can work to change your feeling by engaging in a different behavior. If you seek to be happy, perhaps seeing a good movie will help. Or cognitively, you can think back to a funny experience with your pet and change the sad thoughts, like "I will never be able to live without him/her" to "my pet is in a better place and is no longer suffering." Further, you can say I really enjoyed my time with him/her and when I am ready, I will acquire a new pet. This method can help you naturally grieve for a loss.

If depressed feeling relates to being overwhelmed with stresses and pressures, such as health, finances, job, and relationships, you can work on the initial change of this state by doing a fun activity (behaviorally explained in the next chapter), or work to address your areas of stress by changing these life areas. Continuing to work at a job you hate will not make you feel any better, whereas sending out resumes and applying for new positions and eventually obtaining a better job will make you feel better.

As another negative example, continuing to spend more money than you earn by living your life in debt (i.e., living beyond your means) with no perceived way out will continue to make you feel stressed and depressed. By addressing the real problems and realizing there are other solutions, you can begin to gain more control over your life. This model can help you towards not just short-term change in your life, but long term as well. Is there a feeling driving you to spend money? Can you process this feeling, or at least acknowledge it? What kind of plan can you realistically come up with that will validate your feelings yet honor yourself to make you feel good

17

about getting out of debt? This is how to apply the ABC's by identifying the problem area and creating a realistic solution.

In summary, life is full of contrasts and these are not necessarily bad. By recognizing the differences in your feeling states and accepting them, you can work towards gaining more control over your feelings and your life. As contrasts continue to play a large part in life, you can accept the feeling states you enjoy, change the ones you do not like, and obtain more control over this process as you approach greater mental wellbeing. Additionally, as you do this and get experience with recognizing how you process your feelings, you will become increasingly efficient in addressing your feelings and, over the long haul, will be more effective in your daily life interactions because you have gained control over your experiences. This, in the end, really pays you dividends if you are able to initially put in the work to address the extremes and come up with a manageable solution.

III. BEHAVIOR

Behavior is a central tenet in this model to effect change. If one changes their behavior consistently, they are better able to manage their mental health and problematic symptoms. *Webster's Dictionary* defines behavior as "the actions or reactions of a person or animal in response to external or internal stimuli." What is interesting about this definition is the focus on "actions or reactions." It seems within the definition of behavior that the main point is whether an individual is proactive or reactive. I find this point interesting because this is exactly my focal point. Take charge of your life by being active and taking action instead of letting symptoms take hold of you. It is very difficult to get motivated when you're feeling tired, low, sad, or depressed, but that's the time to become active, to push yourself and try extra hard to keep yourself out of the deep throws of a full-blown depression (or anxiety attack).

Focusing on and controlling your behavior thus becomes a significant way to manage your life and your mental health. In addition, there are multiple times or points where one can intervene prior to a full-blown depressive episode. Those points are discussed in more detail in the INTERVENTIONS CHAPTER.

BEHAVIORAL ACTIVITIES

The following list represents a large range of BEHAVIORAL ACTIVITIES that can be utilized to reduce depressive behavior and keep positive and active:
1) Taking a bath
2) Lighting scented candles

3) Getting a massage
4) Relaxing by laying out in the sun
5) Taking a sauna or steam bath
6) Having quiet evenings
7) Collection activities (coins, stamps, baseball cards, comics, shells, model building, etc.)
8) Reading magazines, newspapers, or books
9) Doing crossword puzzles
10) Making a list of tasks
11) Writing diary entries, letters or a journal
12) Planning a vacation
13) Going on vacation
14) Traveling abroad or in the United States
15) Going on a date
16) Having lunch with a friend; talking to a friend
17) Spending an evening with good friends
18) Sitting at a sidewalk cafe
19) Attending a movie in the middle of the week
20) Going camping
21) Walking in the woods or by the waterfront or in town
22) Going to the beach
23) Flying a kite
24) Fishing
25) Going swimming, waterskiing, jet skiing
26) Sailing, snorkeling
27) White-water canoeing
28) Paintball
29) Going to the mountains
30) Going on a picnic
31) Going to a museum
32) Listening to music

33) Buying music
34) Watching TV
35) Talking on the phone
36) Listening to the radio
37) Laughing
38) Listening to others
39) Having discussions with friends
40) Discussing books, poems, or articles
41) Playing cards or board games
42) Playing a musical instrument
43) Having a political discussion
44) Playing video games
45) Having an aquarium
46) Going to an aquarium or zoo
47) Visiting a National park
48) Photography
49) Seeing a play or concert
50) Exercising
51) Jogging, walking
52) Running track
53) Yoga
54) Playing golf
55) Playing soccer
56) Playing volleyball
57) Playing softball
58) Going to a batting or driving range
59) Miniature golf
60) Bowling
61) Shooting pool
62) Skating
63) Skiing

64) Tennis
65) Going horseback riding
66) Hiking
67) Hunting
68) Doing woodwork
69) Acting
70) Painting
71) Gardening
72) Cleaning
73) Arts and crafts
74) Watching children play
75) Going to a spectator sport (auto or horse racing, professional sports)
76) Watching boxing or wrestling
77) Taking ballet or tap dancing
78) Dancing
79) Flirting
80) Wearing sexy clothes
81) Sex
82) Playing with animals
83) Riding a motorbike or go-cart
84) Driving
85) Eating (favorite foods)
86) Doodling
87) Sightseeing
88) Shopping
89) Buying household gadgets
90) Buying clothes
91) Splurging on a gift for yourself or a nice meal
92) Buying or selling stocks
93) Buying gifts

94) Working on your car or bicycle
95) Meeting new people
96) Planning a day's activities
97) Entertaining
98) Recalling past parties or memories
99) Seeing and/or showing photos
100) Having family get-togethers
101) Planning parties
102) Going out to dinner or breakfast
103) Cooking
104) Community service or volunteering (Big Brother/Big Sister)
105) Searching iTunes
106) Surfing the web
107) Getting coffee or tea or a Slurpee
108) And even sleeping

As you can see, there are many activities to choose from. Why are these activities important? They are important because they focus on pleasurable, positive experiences. In reviewing the list, we notice items or activities that may have been forgotten or never even thought of. This list is meant to help you find positive and meaningful activities to spend time on in order to prevent yourself from falling further into depression. These activities are meant to be a prophylactic, meaning that they are meant to prevent you from getting into a "deep down funk." By themselves these activities cannot cure clinical depression, but are meant to help you get out of your "funk" to prevent further depression. Clinical depression is more thoroughly defined in the chapter on Interventions for Depression, but suffice to say it's a deeper, less transient feeling state of a low mood that requires professional help and intervention by a trained mental health provider like a social worker, psychiatrist or psychologist. It typically involves a change in sleep, appetite, and energy level.

EXERCISE

Within this list of activities, various forms of exercise appear because exercise has multiple benefits, including obtaining a cardiovascular workout that is healthy for your heart and muscles. By exercising, you are working on addressing your physical health and we all know that our physical health is connected to our mental health. For example, going to the gym and incorporating this routine into your daily life can reduce stress, improve the functioning of your body, and enable you to be more productive at work. You might increase your life productivity because you are focusing on the balance of your mind and body.

Other benefits of exercise include the opportunity to socialize and meet new people, blow off some steam, or be part of a group. Our identity is shaped by not only who we are and what we do, but by the people we are involved with and the activities we participate in. Involvement with a recreational sports team might allow you to form an identity related to the team and the outcome of what that team can accomplish. It's a way to not only socialize and exercise, but also to become part of something bigger than ourselves. It feels great to win a game when you were able to help a teammate accomplish something or when together as a team you were able to function at a higher level than as separate individuals. Extend this feeling to winning a championship in tennis, softball, volleyball, or basketball and the satisfaction can be even better.

Simple exercises to strengthen your body can really bring together your life and keep you feeling good. Let's extend this daily gym routine of working out regularly, three or five times a week, and over time, you not only are feeling good, but also are looking good. You start to change your cognitions or thoughts about yourself. Instead of saying "I am fat," you begin to say, "I am looking good" or "I feel really good about myself." Don't think this is realistic? Try it. You will see that once you stick to a routine and put the time in, the rewards can be fantastic.

This exercise routine can lead to greater self-esteem. Simply stated, it means you will feel better about yourself and be confident in your abilities. When you look in the mirror, you will smile and be proud of your accomplishments. An inner confidence or aura will develop and others might begin to react differently toward you.

There is a great movie starring Tim Allen entitled *Joe Somebody* about a man whose wife is leaving him, who gets into an altercation with a bully at work, and decides he is tired of being taken advantage of. He reflects on his life, understands that he did not like the way he handled the altercation and works to strengthen himself in multiple ways. This includes physical exercise, taking a self-defense class, and changing his perspective on life. While he begins to initiate that self-change, he improves his self-esteem and self-worth and others around him react to him in a different manner.

The point of this very entertaining movie is that you can strengthen your life and yourself, which in-turn makes others react or treat you differently. By focusing on yourself as an individual and working to improve yourself, you can obtain real, tangible dividends. Physical, mental, and emotional areas can all be addressed and by using this simple model to guide you in life, you can more readily identify your reactions and the areas you can work on to change.

RELIGION/SPIRITUALITY

I purposely left out religion or spirituality because this can also be a stronghold in one's life. Having spirituality or religion in one's life can also affect your mental health, giving us a place to turn when we don't have answers and providing guidance in various ways. Through religion, we are better able to make sense out of our world. By combining the power we have over our lives (we are not powerless) with some spiritual or religious principles and guidance, we can live better lives.

Religion and spirituality provide a few additional benefits outside of life direction. It provides socialization and community. Sometimes it brings comfort through positive childhood memories or during a stressful time in your life when kinship and brotherhood are comforting. It allows us to be more complete individuals, to share our lives, and feel connected.

In general, we seek out a connection, to feel understood, and to be among similar brethren. By being involved with others within a religious atmosphere, we can have our lives enriched by others and make other people's lives better. This connection can also stimulate additional group activities like community service, support for projects or life goals. In its entirety, socialization and fellowship can protect against the isolatory draw of depression and mental illness.

Taken together, the various behavioral activities outlined provide some relief, meaning and guidance in de-stressing our lives.

EXTREMES

This topic covers the extremes of behavior and the need to not only find balance, but to maintain a balanced life. It's important to find a middle ground in life in various areas. For example, making the daily grind of life easier can simply be a matter of choice. Is getting that cheaper airfare at a distant airport worth the extra stress of driving a longer distance and exposing yourself to more traffic and more headaches? Is waiting for that cheaper flight worth the hassle and energy of worrying about obtaining the flight to a destination where you have to be at a certain time?

In life, there are numerous costs and benefits to daily events and we usually have various choices. How we decide to live our lives by the daily choices that we make can have a tremendous impact on our quality of life. Whenever you choose an extreme choice in life, there are usually consequences. The old adage "the greater the risk, the greater the reward" holds true in some cases, but in our mental health typically that isn't the case.

Within all the behavior or activities, including exercise and religion, there are extremes in both quantity and quality. One can go to the gym and work out seven days a week or one day a year. These extremes on the continuum of behavior are characterized in terms of quantity. It is the same thing with a church or temple, where an individual may attend every single service, only services on the major holidays, or not attend any religious functions at all. This is the continuum of extremes. On a scale of 1 to 10, with the left side (1) representing hardly any activity, and the right side (10) being extreme amounts of activity, it's important to find a middle ground or happy medium.

Examples of extremes in behavior in terms of quality might be the difference between chopped steak and the finest filet mignon, or between sex that has become commonplace and ecstatic, mind-blowing intercourse. Other comparisons might include the difference between like and love, attraction and lust, or annoyance and hate. These represent the extremes on the continuum of the quality of a behavior or the feelings attached to the behavior.

PSYCHOLOGICAL IMPLICATIONS

Taken together, differences in both quality and quantity can affect our mental health and balance. Let's face it; the difference between a local flight of less than two hours and a flight across the country for six hours is a big difference in quantity. Sitting in first class or coach is a difference in quality. What is the big difference? These cases are a lesser example of extremes in behavior. Is the difference between a local flight and an intercontinental flight noticeable? Who wants to be doing any activity continuously for eight, ten or twelve hours, especially sitting? I have racked my brain and cannot think of any activity that I would like to do for more than ten hours straight and that even includes sex and sleep.

This is the extreme example of an activity. Something more tangible in our daily lives to focus on is food and how problems may ensue. Extremes in consumption of food can have very deleterious effects. If you have a diet of high cholesterol and fatty foods, you place yourself at a considerable health risk. But what natural or external forces help shape this diet? Who were your role models? What if you were raised eating this type of food and did not know there was anything wrong with it? What if eating certain foods was associated with positive memories in childhood? Or perhaps negative memories? What if you have internalized all the advertising we are bombarded with on television so that you believe that you must eat Domino's pizza, Crispy Crème or Dunkin Donuts, or McDonalds? What if you have a psychological need to consume greasy, fatty foods to make you feel better? What if this helps fill the gaps or holes in your life, perhaps to make you feel full, although you live an empty life, paralleling shopping or spending more money than you have?

Can psychological needs push one to have excessive or extreme behavior? To feel good about oneself, does a person need to constantly be involved in a relationship with someone? What about constantly having sex or overcompensating in a relationship by continually giving into another's needs at the cost of your own needs? What about working excessively, like 60, 80, or 100 hours a week. What does that do? Does it help? Not really. It enables one to avoid looking at their life, not only to taking an inventory of the things they like, but also to possibly change and shape the things they dislike.

29

Our behavior has a deeper, richer meaning than we think we know. By understanding the cause of our overeating, undereating, overworking, being unemployed, over-shopping, being self-reliant or totally dependent, we not only gain insight but also can make deeper changes. Having the tools like the ABC's to change behavior through identifying the different contributors can only improve your life.

You can also break down the sequence of specific behaviors and analyze the sequential course of your behavior but this will not lead to change. Although you will have the necessary tools to change your behavior, it will be up to you to explore the reasons for your behavior and make important modifications.

In psychological terms, it's the difference between using a cognitive-behavior (CBT) approach that focuses on your current behavior and how to change it, versus reviewing your past to gain an understanding of how it influences your current and future behavior. In other words, this is the difference between an ahistorical approach like CBT or a historical approach like psychoanalytic or psychodynamic therapy. The difference in approach is where you both discount your past and do not take it into account, or you recognize your history and its contributions to your current life.

Can psychological needs push one to have excessive or extreme behavior? The answer is yes. How can one address the extremes of behavior? Does one have to address the psychological needs? The question is rhetorical, the answer is atheoretical.

BEHAVIORAL ABC'S

Another set of ABC's, namely within BEHAVIOR, can be thought of as the antecedents, the behavior itself, and consequences to this action. The diagram below highlights the pathway of the behavioral chain of events.

A---------→---------→-------B--------→-------------→----------C
Antecedent   Behavior   Consequences

Most often, a behavioral event has something that comes before it and something that comes after it. It's like a behavioral chain of events with the segments being labeled the antecedents and consequences respectively. Why is this so important? It's important because being aware of the antecedents and your reactions to the behavior, or the reactions of others, can lead to change or reshaping behavior.

For example, if you want to quit smoking—not an unusual behavior to want to change—you might begin by identifying the antecedents to your craving. These might include stress at the workplace or simply the desire to have a cigarette after a meal. Thus, you have now identified what happens to set off the chain of behavior.

Outside of your behavior and the environment you're in, there are physical dependency needs associated with cigarette smoking like nicotine dependency. Realizing both aspects are related to behavioral change, you might try to use a chewing gum that releases nicotine or a nicotine patch. To maintain this change, you should try to come up with alternative behaviors to take the place of your typical behavior or response.

For instance, when you get stressed at work, rather than reaching for a cigarette you might want to go for a walk or get a cool beverage. The more specific your intervention, the more likely it will lead to an extinction of that behavior. For example, drinking a cold drink is very similar to cigarette smoking in that you are using your hand, raising it to your mouth, and placing something into your mouth. By leaving the stressful environment, like taking a walk to get a cold drink, you are substituting an equivalent behavior to the action of smoking a cigarette where you walk to a smoking section.

Another example, near and dear to my heart, is lactose intolerance. An individual suffering from this physical illness has trouble digesting the sugar lactose. Consumption of dairy products, such as rich creamy ice cream, has been associated with the lactose related problems of gastro-intestinal symptoms. These symptoms include bloating, nausea, diarrhea, congestion, indigestion, and stomach aches. Even though this is an under-diagnosed illness, symptoms are painful and distressing but they tend to be short lasting.

If we think about our behavioral chain, we can quickly isolate the consumption of rich creamy ice cream as the culprit to physical pain. Let's look at what happened right before you went to get ice cream. Maybe its summer and you were hot and began to crave ice cream. Or you were stressed at work and went for some relief with a scoop of ice cream, not realizing that this would upset your stomach. I do not mean to dissect every behavior we have, but to show these examples to identify ways we can make lasting behavioral change.

In the prior example, it's a hot day and you went for ice cream. Typically, this is a non-changeable antecedent behavior, right? Wrong! There are many hot days and there are many other behaviors besides eating ice cream. On this occasion, feeling hot, you decided to get some ice cream to cool you down and enjoyed its good taste, but afterwards had the consequence of having an upset stomach or diarrhea. The rich and creamy ice cream is loaded with calories and cholesterol, which also might not be that healthy for you. Under normal circumstances, moderation is okay as long as you're not hypertensive, diabetic, or have heart problems, but there could be long-term consequences to your behavioral CHOICES.

I clearly write CHOICES because we all have choices, whether or not to do a certain behavior or whether or not to eat a certain food. Sometimes we might feel like we do not have choices or we seem unaware of our choices, but in life we do have choices. In the above example, our choices could have included ice water, iced coffee, sorbet, frozen yogurt, gazpacho (cold soup), getting into the shade, going for a swim, staying in an air conditioned room, and taking a cold shower or bath. Plenty of choices, right?

So why did we chose ice cream? It's obvious, because it tastes good. Maybe it evoked childhood memories of the ice cream man and you wanted to relive your childhood or reminisce, or you just craved something sweet. What if it was chocolate ice cream and you wanted a little pick-me-up from the caffeine and sugar? We all have the ability to identify the reasons behind our actions and to determine if changing behavior is worth it. Maybe you can take an enzyme-inhibiting pill to address your lactose intolerance because you simply love ice cream. Taking it to the extreme, perhaps you enjoy visiting the dentist and feel the most pleasurable way to get there is with new cavities, thanks to the sugar rich ice cream. Whatever your reasons for this behavior and maintaining your behavior, you can be empowered to make a decision. Remember, not doing anything is still making a choice.

In this discussion, my point was to identify the specific antecedents in your behavioral choices, the consequences to your actions, logical alternatives including options or other ways to cope, and the options in making behavioral changes that take into account the series of factors involved in your behavioral choice. Getting a cold drink instead of smoking takes into account the physical action of using your hand to put something in your mouth. This aspect of the BEHAVIORAL ABC'S (Antecedent, Behavior, and Consequence), the physical act of putting something in your mouth, can lead to an understanding of your BEHAVIOR which can help you determine an appropriate CHOICE.

With CHOICE, it is important to identify the continuum of behavior or behavioral options. Again, the concept of CONTRAST can help elucidate CHOICES. Contrasting behavioral choices can be highlighted in two ways in terms of quantity and quality. Quantity means the frequency in terms of excessive or not at all. It's the difference between working out at a gym seven days a week for five hours a day or not working out at all during the entire year.

The concept of CONTRAST is very important because you can choose a behavior that is incongruent (i.e., a healthy behavior) to a more destructive behavior. Choosing a healthy behavior really means that you avoid an unhealthy one. For example, if you're feeling sad and depressed and think an alcoholic drink might make you feel better, if you chose to exercise instead—simply stated since you realistically cannot do both—this healthy behavior can help you avoid an unhealthy behavior. Or, instead of choosing an alcoholic beverage to meet your psychological need AND quench your thirst, you chose an alternative beverage that is not as harmful, like a milkshake, glass of juice or a fruit smoothie.

Another example of a healthy versus unhealthy behavior is staying out until the wee hours of the morning when you work full-time instead of getting a good night's rest. Or simply sitting at home and watching TV instead of going to the gym when you know you need the exercise. On the continuum of activity, if one is active, one cannot be inactive.

Extending this rationale to our daily lives, if you eat healthy and exercise, you probably will not gain weight. If you go to see a good comedy movie, you probably will not be in a mood to start a fight or cry. These behaviors are contrasting or incongruous and if you are practicing one of these behaviors, you will automatically be preventing the other.

As with AFFECT, using the continuum of behavior as a guide, when you're on one extreme on the behavioral continuum, as you shift toward the other side of the continuum, your behavior will change toward your goals. On the other hand, if you were satisfied with your behavior, there would be no need to change it.

The QUALITY of a behavior also has contrasting attributes. For instance, you can either eat a greasy hamburger or filet mignon in a fine restaurant. This experience or activity of eating differs tremendously in quality. While there is value in each separate experience, because sometimes we just want to have a really good burger, at other times we want to have a fine, elegant meal with a great piece of beef that is cooked to perfection.

The focus is on the outcome of your behavioral choice and you are in control of choosing the type of behavior that leads to a predetermined outcome. This is the most important and central aspect to implementing the ABC's: identifying where your behavior stands on the continuum and shifting your stance (behavior) toward the outcome you are seeking. Although it sounds easy enough, implementing this type of change can take motivation, courage, strength, will power, and perseverance.

If you are able to implement a change and be committed to this change, you can improve your mental health and life. When you're in the process of changing after precontemplation and contemplation, you move to what Pliska and DeClemente describe as the action stage. While action is needed, it is important to find a balance with your Affect, Behavior, and Cognitions. In a way, a favorable position would be to straddle the fence as you adhere to moderation in your search for a happy medium.

IV. COGNITIONS

Cognitions are our thoughts or thinking processes associated with our daily life. We are constantly thinking and sometimes our thoughts can affect or control our mood and emotions. As indicated in the model, our cognitions play a large part in our mental health. When an individual has negative cognitions such as "I am no good," "I am worthless," or "I am a failure," these can be internalized and repeated over and over until one believes them. In this way, they affect our mental health in a most negative way.

This focus on our negative behavior is called brooding or perseveration, where an individual has trouble letting go of a thought and dwells on it. When an individual fixates on such a thought, freeing himself or herself from that thought is difficult. To make matters worse, not being able to move on to other subjects can worsen their mood. For example, if one continually thinks, "I will never pass this test in school" during the exam, it will increase their anxiety to a very unhealthy level. Or if they think, "I am scared to drive over bridges," this will produce heightened symptoms of anxiety while driving.

Cognitions are self-thoughts we have about ourselves or our environment and when taken separately, they are very healthy. We typically have many positive thoughts throughout the day, from general everyday observations, to reminiscing, to planning for the future. We can also think negatively, brooding on a mistake we made, something stupid we said, something we forgot or did not do, or some missed opportunity. Cognitions can become unhealthy when negative and continually repeated.

Once again, the common theme of moderation in our thought patterns is very important. For example, what if you only think about your upcoming mortgage payment once and then forget to pay it. A lack of thought or cognition may be detrimental. On the other extreme, constantly thinking about and worrying over your mortgage payment might be very unhealthy. If thinking about paying your mortgage motivates you to pay it or gets you to work harder to earn more money to cover the expense, this may be healthy, but if these constant thoughts make you anxious and depressed, it can become very unhealthy.

If you had a disease, would brooding over it continually be helpful? How do you determine moderation? To quote Donna Summer, how do you know when "enough is enough?"

To use the classic psychologist answer, "it depends." If thinking about something takes up all your time or prevents you from doing things, then that can be unhealthy. As a rule of thumb, you need to find a balance between thinking or forgetting about something. To avoid thinking about a topic or doing an action can be unhealthy. Remember, thoughts usually come before action, so one needs to think about topics before working towards changing the behavior. If you constantly think about a topic, to the point of being incapacitated and stuck, then that becomes just as unhealthy as avoiding a topic or thought.

Let's look into problematic thought patterns and construct some solutions. If you constantly think about a topic or problem that is currently on your mind to the point of being unproductive, what can you do about it?

One solution to stop thinking about the problem includes scheduling a time to think about the problem. Perhaps you can do it at 10PM, right before you go to bed for say half an hour. Sounds corny? Try it. By using this technique, the process validates your concern about the problem and allows you to better manage your time by scheduling a time to worry or "work" on this problem. It is almost like a job where you have certain times to do certain things. You log onto you computer when you begin work, or you go to lunch between 12 and 1PM. This teaches us to schedule in time to deal with our problematic thoughts. It makes us more structured, organized, and most importantly, **in control** of our problems.

Another technique is to write the problem down so that you gain control or mastery over it. This way you are again validating that it is an important concern but also substantiating that there is a time and a place for everything, and most importantly to make you realize that this problem or idea will not control your life.

A simple solution is to prepare a "cognitive to-do list." Think about it. We have plenty of behavioral to-do lists where things need to get done, so what is wrong with creating a cognitive to-do list? When was the last time you had free time, let alone set aside free time to think? It is very important for your mental health to have time to yourself, and if you are constantly worrying about a problem or idea, maybe by "scheduling it in" you can free yourself to do other things.

DICHOTOMOUS THINKING

We have covered the quantity of thoughts including the repetitiveness of or absence of thoughts, but we must also be concerned about the quality of thoughts. Dichotomous thinking is simply thinking in an either-or manner, sort of like only seeing two solutions. This type of thinking has been labeled black or white thinking versus seeing different options or experiencing the grey. We can think of it as a polarized type of thinking. You are either on one side of the fence or the other.

Examples of dichotomous thinking include yes or no thinking versus maybe; right or wrong instead of it depends; or "either this or that." Thinking in a yes or no manner is juvenile and childlike, especially when adults only use dichotomous thoughts. In life, there are many questions that have no answers or the answers are complicated. Psychologists are trained to identify and examine an individual's thought quality, but when people use a dichotomous organization to interpret life's events and conceptualize their environment in this way, it can lead to a tremendous disadvantage in negotiating everyday tasks with others.

Although people don't necessarily talk or think about our thought quality, people who use a dichotomous style are rigid in their thinking and can be described as "intellectually immature" and inflexible. This concept is so vital to our mental health because our cognitive processes comprise a huge portion of our day since we are almost always thinking and therefore can affect almost every interaction. By using this undeveloped thought organization, we curb ourselves of the many options that exist not only in our thoughts but also in our behavior and life.

Extending this concept, there exist a continuum of thoughts just like there is a continuum of behavior, and there are a variety of options we have when we are unrestricted or creative in our thought processes. By using a creative style, this type of thinking provides the vehicle to more options and choices and, by comparison, is more flexible.

As an example, let's say you are waiting for someone to pick you up on a date, and that someone is late. You then receive a phone call that cancels your date with some type of excuse. Someone who has a restricted way of thinking might personalize the excuse and think it was solely because of "them." They might think that the person either likes me or does not like me and therefore will not go on a date with me. This is dichotomous thinking. If they have low self-esteem, they might think, "who would want to date me, I am a loser, and I am ugly."

Alternatively, a person with an unrestricted or unconstrained cognitive set or flexible thinking might say to themselves, "they were busy and I understand that sometimes dates are canceled, and that it is not personal." Another person might say, "maybe this person is unsure about going on a date with me" because we need to get to know each other better in order to make the determination of whether or not we should spend more time together and socialize.

By thinking through many of the options involved in this dating example—such as they like me, don't like me, it's situational, it's environmental, the cancellation just happened, don't personalize it, or I am so glad we didn't go out so I could get some things done around the house because I was tight on time—this flexibility reflects a much healthier thought process.

As you can see, there are various ways one can perceive situations, and from one's perception reactions flow (affect or feelings). The dichotomous reaction provides limited responses and probably will lead toward the feeling of anger. If one implements or uses a flexible approach, a variety of outcomes or reactions are possible because they are couched with more understanding of the situation and potential circumstances around the situation. Instead of the environment, such as a potential date, acting upon the person, the person is acting upon their environment. They are able to maintain control and balance. In this example, you are better able to be free to make alternative plans rather than be bogged down by a change of plans.

Cognitive flexibility also comes into play in multiple situations, from hassles in your daily life to major changes that happen during your life. If you are driving and have to change your route because of traffic, being flexible might allow you to change your schedule and maximize your time.

Let's say that a route is blocked on your way home. Being flexible, instead of going directly home, you remember you have errands to run and although a little out of the way, they need to get done. So you might go and pick up your dry cleaning, get gas, and go to the bank and by the time you finish, the traffic clears up. The opposite of this response or "flexibility" is that you would sit in traffic, increase your frustration, irritation and blood pressure, and then come home in a bad mood, not feeling a sense of accomplishment for completing errands. This bad mood could lead to a negative interaction with your significant other or your children and snowball into more problems. Instead, the trip takes the same amount of time because you avoided the traffic and by not wasting time, you were able to knock off a few things that needed to get done and ended up being happy about your accomplishments.

Another way to shape your thinking, in the same "stuck in traffic situation" is to get on the cell phone and make that important phone call or catch up with a friend. Although this is multi-tasking, you are being versatile by making the most out of your time and not focusing on the negative. You are actively shaping or changing what you are focusing on in terms of your thoughts. You are avoiding thinking about the negative aspects of being stuck in traffic by actively doing something else or thinking about positive things. It seems like this solution is "busying yourself up," but in reality it is focusing your thoughts and energies in a positive direction, using the continuum of cognitions (and activities) to help you cope with a semi-difficult situation.

Multi-tasking or flexibility is not the solution to all of life's quandaries, but when you are able to be flexible and think creatively, you are able to come up with quick solutions to temporary problems. Additionally, employing the cognitive triad of the model (ABC's) with the continuum of thoughts allows you to improve the overall quality of your daily existence and can lead to a more satisfying life.

To elaborate on using a flexible approach, a few great examples come from the world of sports. In almost any sport, great athletes are balanced and flexible. For those who know basketball, there is a basic stance called a 3-point stance. In this stance, you have 3 options. Visualize the basketball passed to you and you catch it. Your three options include dribbling the ball, passing the ball, or shooting the ball.

Typically, the 3-point stance involves bending your knees with your feet a shoulder's width apart and maintaining a very flexible stance where you can go in any direction you choose. If you dribble the ball and stop dribbling, you limit your options and now drop down to having only 2 options (pass or shoot).

Let's look at tennis. When you are receiving a serve, your weight is shifting and you are in a balanced position so you can react and go in any direction. Same thing with fielding a baseball; you want to get low to the ground with a low center of gravity and be in balance when you catch the ball. By being balanced prior to the play, you have the widest variety of options at your disposal. With hitting a baseball, you need to be balanced so you can quickly shift your weight and make the determination in a split second whether or not you will attempt to hit the ball.

These examples point to the importance of flexibility and balance. These principles are very useful when applied to cognitive flexibility or exploring the continuum of thoughts in terms of both quantity and quality. The concepts of balance and flexibility will also be more fully discussed in the BALANCE chapter.

V. STRUCTURE

Structure is the daily scheduled activities one creates in their lives to provide stability to each day. Structure is very important because it provides predictability. In a way, it's a routine one can follow to add consistency and balance to one's life.

Having a functional schedule in your life provides a continuity that makes it easier to determine factors that begin to affect your mental health because stressors outside of your daily structure can be readily identified. Additionally, most people thrive from a structured environment because they can improve their skills on daily tasks and focus additional energies on things outside of that structure. In this way, predictability helps ensure manageability and by association improved mental health.

In other words, structure means an organized regimen that you follow in daily life. It begins well before your daily activities. For instance, if you have a regular job and work 9 to 5 with specific responsibilities and you normally go to lunch between 12 and 1, then that is part of your daily structure. Prior to coming to work, you have to wake up and can eat breakfast. Your structure typically begins before that because you need to go to sleep. It might begin at 10 or 11PM when you go to sleep and continues when you wake up, go to the bathroom, brush your teeth, shower, get dressed, have breakfast, and commute to work. This daily work schedule provides structure and if you incorporate your three meals a day into your life, you now begin to see how organized or structured the days really are.

The importance of structure relates to helping you address the daily needs of the workday and home life while taking into account your mental health needs. When you change your structure, you begin to see why it's so important to have consistency in your life. A readily identifiable change in structure that most people can relate to provides a good example. Let's say you are married, have children and work a regular job from 9 to 5. After work, since your day was stressful, you seek a way to relax. You decide to go out with your buddies and get a "drink" early in the week.

When describing a "drink," there are typically only a few types of beverages: caffeinated, alcoholic, or non-caffeinated. We will discuss the G rated version of the story and say that you and a few buddies met up and had some coffee (for those fruit juice smoothie lovers out there, I am sorry).

The conversation goes well, you're entertained and you also have what I like to call a mini "bitch session." Time passes as you continue to reminisce or just "shoot the shit." As time passes, it becomes late at night before you drive home to your wife and children. By the time you get home and do a few things as you get ready for bed, it's late and past your "structured" bedtime.

Now the fun part begins as you try to fall asleep. You are unable to do so and, feeling restless, you begin to toss and turn but just can't get comfortable enough to relax and fall asleep. Maybe you were stimulated by all the conversation or by noticing how other people enjoyed each other's company, especially with the opposite sex. Whatever it is, you seem overstimulated, on edge, and have difficulty falling asleep.

As your alarm goes off the next morning, you groggily try to get yourself going by taking a shower and doing all of the other morning rituals and arrive to work a few minutes late. Without a good night's rest, you seem a bit out of sorts at your job. Additionally, one of the projects you've been working on becomes particularly difficult and you're unable to complete it during the day. Feeling "spent" as the day comes to a close, you again feel like you need a break and want to have some relaxation after another difficult day. Since you had such an enjoyable time with your friends the previous night, you decide to call the fellas up for another evening out.

The same results happen again. Although you are entertained and enjoy the companionship of your friends, by coming home late and feeling unsatisfied that you have to work tomorrow, you have trouble sleeping again. If we extrapolate this scenario, a repetition of the same each day to night, more problems continue at work and you get more edgy and become easily annoyed simply because you're not getting enough sleep. This pattern can become a problem because you are unable to get your work done and you now encounter problems at home with your wife. She complains that you are not home enough to help out around the house or with the kids and this causes relationship strife. Your boss also begins to get on you because the quality of your work has gone down, you don't seem to be as focused, and you constantly arrive late. If these problematic behaviors continue, you might be headed for unemployment and divorce.

What is causing all these problems? Is it simply drinking coffee or alcohol? The answer is more complicated than a simple no, but the predicament can be thought of in simple terms. By analyzing what went wrong, we identify problems in structure and also the previously discussed ABC's of behavior, namely the antecedent, behavior, and consequence as well as the continuum of behavior or need for moderation versus extremes.

Structurally, needing a break from life is a <u>symptom</u> of the problem, which is further exacerbated by the use of a night or two out with friends and the use of a stimulant like coffee with caffeine or alcohol. When you consume large amounts of caffeine, a potential side effect can be sleep difficulties and also frequent urination because caffeine is both a stimulant and a diuretic. By drinking coffee in the late afternoon and evening, the body had trouble metabolizing the caffeine fully and the resultant side effect was difficulty falling asleep.

If we also take into account the need for moderation or less extremes on the continuum, as the rule of thumb states, excessive use of coffee or caffeine represents an extreme type of behavior and can cause problems. By going out more than what would be described as a healthy use of free time, and despite using this coping mechanism of drinking coffee with friends till late at night, it still created problems.

As psychologists, we often try to identify if a behavior causes "clinically significant problems" or if they cause problems in multiple areas in your life leading to difficulties. In this example, it seemed that the man was on his way to such difficulties and hopefully will be able to find healthier, alternative coping mechanisms.

The problems in this example included difficulties with the job, the spouse and not seeing his children. The above is the G rated version. Imagine changing the scenario where excess alcohol was used. Domestic violence, problems with the law like getting a DUI (driving while intoxicated), or health problems can become distinct possibilities. In this example, the problem was approaching clinical significance because of his work and marital problems.

Let's also not forget how the person might be feeling while undergoing these self-inflicted changes. Self-inflicted means that the person actively behaved in such a manner[1] that it led to these negative outcomes. This person might begin to feel depressed, relative to a few troubled areas in his life.

First, we know that when sleep patterns are interrupted, depression can emerge. It is also evident that life problems, such as work or marital troubles, can lead to depression, and the combination of these areas might exacerbate the feelings of depression.

From this extrapolated example, it seems that the coping he used of going out with his buddies was more an escape technique of leaving life and the demands of work, but in the end, negative consequences occurred. The antecedent of drinking and getting to bed late was probably due to feeling bored, tired, or lacking a connection at home or at work. These represent some of the feelings involved in the problem and in order to make a change we can also focus on the behaviors.

Maybe some job difficulties led the person to feel isolated and thus he sought some type of connection or reconnection. Or maybe there were difficulties with the family and marriage and he simply did not want to be home. Whatever the cause, the antecedent—a difficult day at the office—led to the behavior of going out with the guys and drinking coffee, which after repeating, led to the consequences of problems with work and spouse.

---

[1] By choosing a certain type of behavior & repeating this behavior even after it led to more problems; the example of alcohol is clearer when someone continues to drink even after numerous family, employment, legal, & social consequences.

As initially indicated, the importance of disregarding our daily structure coupled with the lack of attention to the ABC's of mental health can lead to tribulations in life. To address these areas and improve our lives, we need to apply the ABC's of mental health.

Furthermore, we can include in our daily life the structure of having time to think. This can include a cognitive "to do" list that was previously suggested. We should also incorporate relaxation time into our daily lives.

We all expend energy and get burnt out over time and need to recharge. By incorporating relaxation time into our daily or weekly schedule, we are taking into account our needs and the necessity to take care of them. Just think of it as a necessary break prior to taking the much-needed vacation. The same applies for allocating time to have fun. We need to participate in fun activities in order to balance out all the difficult times.

The examples cited are just a few ways to increase structure. Other ways to increase structure include diet, exercise, discipline, and assertiveness. But everyone does things their own way. For instance, I knew a woman in graduate school who would never do any school work on the weekends. I could never understand how she was able to accomplish this because my weekends were filled with schoolwork. In fact, it was the only time during the week that I had clumps of time to really get into a project.

Amazingly, she was quite clear in her structure and her rationale was that the weekends were the time for her and her family. On the flip side, she was hardly available during the weeknights; one would assume that was when she was getting her work done.

In this example, the woman I mentioned was very disciplined in her time management, which is the essence of structure. It is the same thing with maintaining a diet; you need to have discipline to avoid forbidden foods while maintaining your schedule of exercise. Structure and the input you have in managing your life is of crucial importance because structure can entail most of life and you can control, to some extent, the structure of your life.

The key to success is identifying when there is a problem and then working to change your structure to address future problems. From drinking to daily spending to time management, you have the mechanisms to influence your quality of life once you recognize the issues. You can either work to improve the structure or explore your own individual ABC's.

In terms of mental health, structure comprises your daily existence and by paying full attention to such parts as sleep, exercise and eating, you can avoid "self-created" problems. In addition, part of your structure is in managing your physical ailments. If you have diabetes or hypertension, you need to consistently take your medications and for the greatest benefit, take them at the same time each day. Additionally, if you have depression or bipolar disorder or other ailments that are treated with psychotropic medications, maintaining the intake and levels of medication in your blood is of paramount importance.

In my practice, I have heard so many times of the difficulties that ensued when medication regimens were changed or compromised. The most common example is when a depressed individual takes an antidepressant like an SSRI (selective serotonin reuptake inhibitor) and reports feeling better. After an extended period of time, they stop taking their medications because they were feeling "better."

Unfortunately, antidepressants do not work the same way as headache medication where you take it as needed. It's very important to build up a therapeutic chemical level of the medication in your blood for it to be effective. Typically it takes between 3 to 4 weeks to build up this level, although some people report some benefits within a few days. Alternatively, it is important to taper off the medication in a similar length of time if you would like to stop using it.

It's amazing how people either forget what made them begin to feel better or they don't attribute the salubrious effects to the pill that they were consuming daily. They don't realize that the mechanism of action that led them to feeling better works the other way when the same system of action is stopped from a discontinuation of their medications.

The typical course of time people need to use antidepressants ranges from a minimum of 3 months to an average of 6 months to a year. If you have a history of major depression, it might be beneficial to continue using an antidepressant as long as it maintains its efficacy.

Without going into more depth on what happens when you consume medications, which will be discussed at length in the MEDICATION chapter, let's just say that the neurotransmitters in your brain are altered from the use of the medications over time and when you abruptly discontinue the medications, your body will react. Therefore, just as you built up the medications over time in your body, it's important to taper off the medications to minimize bodily reaction. Once again, the focus is on maintaining the structure that improves your life.

As I conclude this chapter on structure, I want to reiterate that the structure within one's life can prevent serious difficulties or lessen the exacerbation of the current illness or difficulty. I also want to highlight a great point one of my Veterans made about the difference between our foundation and structure.

If you think of a house as an analogy, it is comprised of a foundation and then the structure. More specifically, the foundation is what the structure is built upon, as this lays the groundwork for the completion of the house. Without a solid foundation, the structure of the house will be insignificant. What is important to recognize is the need for a solid foundation. Unfortunately, the focus of this book has not been on your foundation. If your foundation is not that strong, you might need to strengthen it by seeking professional help like that of a psychologist, social worker, psychiatrist, or other mental health professional.

I point out the differences between foundation and structure for the simple reason that this book focuses on our structure, something we are very much in control of. Our foundation has already been laid through our upbringing and is more difficult to change. It is a more long-term edifice, and therefore very difficult to address in the short-term. This book focuses on things we can change, and I feel that our structure is one such item. The other aspects of the ABC model provide for additional areas for change.

Our foundation, and the need to rebuild this foundation, will take more time and work and therefore cannot possibly be addressed in a single book. Again, a poor foundation might be one that proves difficult to build upon. For example, not having "good enough" parenting or not having a mentor in your life where you had someone you could rely upon to develop a trusting relationship can cause foundational problems. Having a good enough mother, father, grandparent, relative, or mentor in your life can be the factor needed to build a strong foundation. In a way, this can be labeled the "concrete" of your life. Without these ingredients, and by living through horrific abuse, the foundation that has been laid might need more serious intervention than can be provided by a self-help book.

In summary, this chapter focused on structure that we can control and change. By having a strong focus on managing your daily life by changing certain patterns to optimize your structure or being assertive to implement change, you can more fully plot out your pathway to mental health. It was from this focus on structure that you are empowered to change your life.

VI. EMPOWERMENT

The previous chapter was about arranging your daily life or structure to better gain control over life and your mental health. In this form of self-empowerment you feel vitalized and in control of your life. You gain the ability to exert control and empowerment becomes the act of you or someone enabling strength and action.

The importance of empowerment in Mental Health is due to the fact that we tend to feel disenfranchised when all of the energy is sucked out of us, leading us to a feeling of hopelessness. Any good intervention in mental health has as a key component invigorating or motivating an individual to feel like they have more control over their lives than they currently believe they have. It also empowers an individual to action, to make changes, and to become more adept at finding solutions to their problems. It involves increasing one's awareness of our options.

From what we know about depression, one major symptom of depression is the inability to see all the options that are available. Depressed individuals tend to have tunnel vision and are unable to see additional solutions to the problem they are currently experiencing that feels overwhelming. Empowering an individual enables them to see other options and make changes. It is a vital feeling to a person's sense of self and power over their environment and difficulties.

When feeling disenfranchised, you might feel like not doing anything. Multiply this feeling by 10 or 100 and that is the feeling some people face when trying to change their lives. It can be very overwhelming, metaphorically like viewing a towering mountain you must climb. Even thinking about ways to proceed is difficult when one believes a task is overwhelming or even impossible. It is exactly at these times when one feels like they cannot proceed, and at such a time is it vital that you become empowered, and are energized to attack the project and be able to persevere through the difficulty. Challenging? Yes, but **not** impossible. It can be quite difficult to get back into the groove, when feeling unable to invest any more time or energy, but the challenge lies in changing your direction and re-motivating oneself.

To begin this challenge, you first have to validate your feelings. What the heck does *validate* your feelings mean? Validating your feelings means making them real, owning them, authenticating them, and supporting these feelings within yourself. It's the ability to say that these are my feelings and that they are valid for the situation I am in, and that it is okay to have these feelings. This is the first step towards re-empowering yourself to change.

The next step towards empowerment is re-motivating yourself or finding your motivation. When a task is daunting, there are a variety of options you can have to work towards a solution as it is normal to see limited options when one is feeling depressed. There are many diagnoses of mental illness where a symptom is tunnel vision or the inability to see options or feeling limited. Keeping this common symptom in mind is very important so that you do not feel overwhelmed or trapped. In fact, it is vital to normalize this response and by doing so, you more readily can adapt to it.

It is easy to begin to feel overwhelmed, lose focus, and not realize that there are other options. The psychological factors that go into losing motivation are many, including reverting back to past behavior because it is more comfortable. One of the biggest factors is feeling that you are in a no-win situation and as a result you begin to feel helpless. This feeling of helplessness is a major warning sign of depression and, as a result, needs to be addressed quickly. I would even go so far as to say that if you are constantly feeling helpless, you should seek out a mental health provider for therapy and medications.

We know from the ABC's, and specifically the cognitive aspects or "C," that one can begin to develop negative thoughts and these thoughts can multiply and create a change in one's mood or mindset over time. For instance, when you start having negative thoughts and are unable to move forward to accomplish a task, and therefore lose your motivation, you might start to feel depressed. As your frustration grows and you feel less in control, your depression might increase. This process again points out how susceptible we are to mind-feeling relationships while also highlighting and encouraging the various lanes we can change or travel to overcome these obstacles.

As you keep in mind the ABC's and the various strategies to address your depression, you can also focus on ways to keep up your motivation. One strategy is to give yourself some time and allow yourself to "sit" at a difficult place. I also use the synonymous term staying with your frustration and by doing so, you learn to just "be in the moment or feeling" and this can really cause you to become more accepting of self.

By the term "sit" I also mean allowing yourself to think about the situation and come up with a solution over time. Trust that as you work through the difficulty and process it, your brain will come to a solution. This is a process of validating your feeling ("you are confused now") while also trusting yourself to come up with a solution. That is one strategy, to stay with your feeling (recognize, identify, and validate or you can extend this process to a simple acronym—RIVER: recognize, identify, validate, explore, reinvent self).

As an example, if you are feeling burnt out from the daily grind, you might seek a mini-vacation or a 3-day weekend. One example might be going to Las Vegas. Individuals go to Vegas to get away and have a good time. They leave their home surroundings and go off into the never-never land of the city of lights.

In Vegas, there is so much going on until the wee hours of night with a very different focus than what you normally have in your hometown. Typically, the focus is on food, fun, entertainment, gambling and drinks, while the usual hubbub that surrounds your work is left behind. Problematically, you risk getting fully involved in this fast-paced lifestyle of alcohol and gambling and late night adventures.

This last point is brought up because sometimes solutions to problems can cause other problems. Life is about choices, so if you needed a break from the daily grind, a quick getaway might be fantastic, just what the doctor ordered. The cost of such a getaway, on the other hand, and specifically to Las Vegas, can be your energy and money. In addition to the late-night oriented schedule you became accustomed to while staying in Sin City, if you are coming from the East Coast, you also have 3 hours of jetlag to deal with. In other words, your schedule or structure has a dramatic shift, so while you take care of your emotional needs and potentially re-energize by getting away and taking a break, your physical needs and body might not adjust so easily to a different time schedule.

Another strategy to extend your motivation is to shift your focus onto a task or area that you can successfully complete with ease. This will help bolster your confidence for the purpose of recharging your mental and emotional energies so that when you are ready to get back into the original difficult task, you will have the energy to match your motivation. This strategy is similar to a distraction technique, except that you are building your confidence by moving forward, in a way trying to keep or build your momentum so that you can continue with your task.

Another strategy employed is to break down tasks into whole part whole (WPW) configurations. By WPW, you look at the whole task, identify the parts that comprise the whole and work on each of the separate parts so that you can accomplish the whole. In other words, you break down each part to make up the whole and complete "parts" of the task. This strategy can be very effective with large, overwhelming tasks (i.e., a dissertation).

As you work on addressing your motivational needs and empowering yourself from emotional difficulties by employing the ABC's, it is also important to recognize your limitations. I use the term limitations to mean the natural course of events, such as the natural progression we all face in our daily battles. Sometimes we are just having an "off" day and when you are having one of these days, you need to recognize it and quite possibly permit yourself to have an "off-day."

This process of recognizing an "off-day" employs the concept of flow. This concept comes from the literature of physical education and engineering where entities are synchronized and working together naturally to produce very strong and positive outcomes. Being inflow as a process is positive, where an individual is productive and things work out. Being **out of**

flow is when obstacle after obstacle comes your way as you try to achieve your goals.

This concept helps you identify when you're "inflow" versus "out of flow" and when you're out of flow, giving yourself permission to be ineffective or "off." It's a way of being kind to yourself while recognizing your own humanity as we "swim upstream." This can make the process of re-motivation a bit easier if you recognize that you might just be having a "bad day" rather than "lost in creativity." It can also help stop the negative cycle of downward thinking where mood and motivation are negatively escalated by placing the lack of progress on yourself instead of simply being "out of flow." The ramifications of the latter rely on an approach versus the self-blame view. By focusing on your approach, you can prevent a negative cycle from beginning and escalating. By giving yourself permission to not always be "on" or perfect, you empower yourself to "get back on the horse" at a future time and thus decrease the probability that you will focus on the negative, which can exacerbate your problems instead of lessening them. This latter concept of flow and your reaction to "bumps in the road" are the psychological ramifications of the ABC model that helps you to become self-empowered.[2] It enables you to avoid escalating negative thoughts or feelings while at the same time giving yourself permission to have an "off-day" and being flexible with yourself.

In summary, the strategies discussed can be used as a heuristic or aid toward increasing your motivation and empower-

---

[2] I use this example because ideally you have empowered yourself to handle your first gut level reactions by using your cognitive strength to help prevent escalation of the negative, and therefore, changing the outcome of very negative and damaging cycles of thought and behavior.

ing yourself to make changes in your life. If these are applied daily, you might find yourself generating more self-power and confidence in your reactions to life, and through increased insight into your reactions, you can better address or control what happens from your responses to "challenges." You can change your typical response to a new, more effective response and thus break the negative cycles.

VII. MEDICATIONS

Medications, plain and simple, are very important if you are suffering. Whether it's an antidepressant, anti-anxiety medication, medications for diabetes or high blood pressure, or mood stabilizers for Bipolar disorder, medically necessary medications are extremely important to life. Without such interventions, people can suffer or even die.

I emphasize medically necessary medications because some people abuse medications, whether it's painkillers (Vicodin or Percocet) or anti-anxiety medications (Xanax). For others, like those suffering from diabetes, medications such as insulin are needed for survival. This same philosophy can be applied for a chronically depressed or mentally ill individual.

As the chapter heading suggests, I would like to focus on the need for medications and then some specific characteristics and side effects of medications. As a quick caveat, although I have worked in Medical Centers for my entire career, I am not a psychiatrist and therefore I do not have a license to prescribe medications. I offer this chapter as guidance for individuals to follow. For those interested in obtaining more specific information about how antidepressants or other medications work, I refer the reader to *Psychotropic Drugs*, 2nd Edition, by Norman Keltner and David Folks, or to *Listening to Prozac* by Peter Kramer.

When I mention medications, and specifically medications for depression, I want to clarify that I am talking about medications to be used with a diagnosis of depression as opposed to a diagnosis of a mood disorder. Mood disorders, sometimes referred to as manic-depression or Bipolar disorder, entail periods of both depression and periods of high energy or grandiosity. These are separate, distinct states that are not typically felt or experienced at the same time. While there are derivatives of this disorder where both symptoms can be experienced simultaneously, like cyclothymic disorder or rapid cycling where an individual cycles between both states quickly, I will discuss a straightforward presentation of Bipolar disorder.

The term Bipolar comes from a person being on two ends of the pole or extremes, either depressed or manic. It's a very fitting term that takes into account both extreme types of behavior. As will become evident, these different types of extreme behaviors, mania and depression, fit very nicely with our past discussion of behavioral extremes.

In order to treat someone with either depression or mania, the medications are set about to reverse the current physical state they are in. If you're too energetic and grandiose, the medications try to modulate and balance you by moving you to the other side of the extreme. If you are depressed and lacking energy and motivation, the antidepressants try to give you more energy and enable you to feel more pleasure in life.

In theory, they work by neurochemically addressing the extreme aspect of the illness and move you back into a balanced state. This movement or mechanism is similar to the previously discussed use of the ABC's where you learn to move yourself from one extreme position to the grey or middle ground. This is exactly what the medications try to do through neurochemical means.

Without getting into to much biomedical detail about how these drugs work, like selective serotonin reuptake inhibitors, suffice it to say that these medications either increase the availability of a neurotransmitter in your brain, slow the reuptake of the neurotransmitter, or reduce the stimulation of the site where the neurotransmitter is received. Most of the medications available act on one or a combination of the four major groups of neurotransmitters. These are the monoamines, cholinergics, neuropeptides, and amino acids.

As you can see from the name monoamines, these neurotransmitters are involved in the class of antidepressants titled the monoamine oxidase inhibitors (MAOIs). The other neurotransmitters differ in their modes of action and where their action takes place. Typically, the neurotransmitters serotonin, dopamine, epinephrine, and norepinephrine are involved in the mechanism of action in the newer antidepressant medications. This includes the class of medications entitled the SSRI's (selective serotonin reuptake inhibitors) as well as the newer NSRI's (norepinephrine and serotonin reuptake inhibitors).

SSRI's are considered by most experts to be the first choice in antidepressant therapy because they produce fewer side effects and are very effective. SSRI's include Prozac (fluoxetine), Luvox (fluvoxamine), Zoloft (sertraline), Celexa (Citalopram), Lexapro (escitalopram oxalate) and Paxil (paroxetine). The NSRI's include Effexor (Venlafaxine), Cymbalta (duloxetine HCL), and Serzone (nefazodone) while another antidepressant, Wellbutrin (bupropion), has some properties of both, but differs because of its activating quality.

Frequent side effects of SSRI's include gastrointestinal complaints, agitation, headaches, insomnia, somnolence, and sexual dysfunction. As you can tell from the list, the potential side effects depend on the person taking the medication because there are quite a few contradictory side effects, like increased lethargy versus increased energy. Even the side effect of sexual dysfunction has contradictory findings because many individuals experience robust orgasmic function with SSRI's. In support of this finding, SSRI's have been prescribed in the treatment of premature ejaculation.

As you try and digest all this information, one might ask, "Why should I use an antidepressant?" My viewpoint on using antidepressants is quite simple, but has changed over time. In the beginning of my training, I was against the use of medications for the treatment of psychological disorders. Over time, as I trained in medical centers, I realized the beneficial effects of psychotropic medications and gradually shifted my position into full support of these medications. The reason for my shift in position was twofold. First, I began to see firsthand the benefits of these medications. Additionally, when used in conjunction with psychotherapy, antidepressants have been proven to strengthen clinical outcomes. In other words, people do better with a combination of treatments because the antidepressants work to energize individuals and allow them to work through their issues. When people are depressed, they usually lack energy, motivation, and concentration to address the things in their life that are bothering them. An antidepressant, when taken properly, works to increase people's energy and decrease the depressive symptoms over time.

The SSRI's need to be taken every day as prescribed, and they have to be continued daily. The reason for the daily use of antidepressants is that in order for this medication to be successful, one has to build up a therapeutic level in their blood. This typically occurs between three to four weeks after continual use. In addition, patients need to maintain the use of the drug so that they can sustain a therapeutic level in their blood.

While some people might gain some benefits by using antidepressants in the first few days, typically it takes two to four weeks. Again, it should be stressed that the medications need to be taken every day, not just when you are feeling depressed. Antidepressants do not work like aspirin, where you take a pill when you are in pain to relieve the pain. Antidepressants and specifically SSRI's need to be taken daily, and usually are taken for a minimum of 4 months, but typically around one year.

The number one reason people are unable to find relief of depression by using an antidepressant is that they did not take the medication daily as prescribed. In addition, the number one reason a person re-experiences depression is because they stopped taking the medication. If you are feeling better after taking an antidepressant for a few months, the best thing you can do is continue taking the medications. If you would like to get off the medications, as most people usually desire, then you should talk to your doctor and have your medication gradually decreased over time. The term for this is tapering, where you begin to decrease the strength or milligrams that you take over time. Just as you had to build up the milligrams or therapeutic effect in your body over time, you need to reduce this level or volume gradually. The danger in abruptly discontinuing your medications is twofold: your body can either react in a negative way to the abrupt stoppage of medications, or you can return to a worsened feeling of depression.

BIPOLAR DISORDER

I had also previously discussed a different depressive disorder, labeled Bipolar disorder. The difference between Bipolar disorder and depression is that people with Bipolar experience the opposite end of the spectrum, or manic type symptoms. While both Bipolar patients and depressed patients can share the symptom of depression, only Bipolar patients experience mania. Because of this danger, people with Bipolar are not typically treated with antidepressants, but are treated with a different class of drugs called mood stabilizers. Lithium or valproate are the most commonly used drugs to treat Bipolar disorder, but antipsychotic and anxiolytic drugs may also be useful in treating actively manic or agitated patients. In addition, Tegretol (carbamazepine) may be useful in treating acute mania.

When treating Bipolar disorder, the drug level needs to be monitored in the patient's blood so that they maintain an appropriate therapeutic range. Sometimes patients require frequent monitoring to avoid falling into either the manic or depressive symptom presentation. In addition, patient's need to watch their hydration levels because dehydration can lead to changing lithium or depokoate levels and other side effects are also monitored to address concerns related to other body functions (white blood cell count, liver, etc.).

BENEFITS OF MOOD STABILIZERS AND ANTIDEPRESSANTS

These medications help people re-engage in social, occupational, and relationship functioning that leads to an improvement in quality of life. For patients suffering Bipolar disorder, these medications help modulate their mood and work to stabilize their mood shifts into a more normalized pattern. In other words, these medications balance the patient out. For some, these medications become a way of life due to the chemical imbalance that they endure. Without taking the appropriate medications as prescribed, these patients can suffer serious consequences.

For more information on the difficulty of managing Bipolar disorder, *The Unquiet Mind* by Kay Redfield Jamison is an excellent read. This book is the perennial description of the constant suffering of Bipolar disorder and the difficulties encountered when one is not properly medicated. It is also a personalized viewpoint of the struggles a Bipolar individual goes through and highlights the difficulties a person faces when beginning a medication to stabilize their mood. This results in the individual not experiencing the "high highs" while also not having the "low lows" and is a major reason Bipolar individuals are resistant to taking a mood stabilizer because they want to continue feeling the "high highs."

As I conclude this chapter, I want to stress the importance not just of the effectiveness of medications in treating depression, but of changing your structure to incorporate medications in your daily life when needed. I also want to highlight that taking a pill every day will not solve all of your problems. Remember, taking an antidepressant or medication will not CHANGE your life or the problems you face daily. This requires more than simply taking a little pill. It requires examining your daily structure, your affect, behavior, cognitions, and your problems and coming up with solutions.

Antidepressants can assist you in gaining control over your life and problems by energizing you to tackle life's problems. More importantly, as antidepressants begin to work and you begin to address your problems, you will begin to see more options and feel more in control over your life.

As will be discovered in the next chapter, I emphasize the importance of communication in dealing with your daily problems. Problems usually occur between individuals when there is no communication or the ideas are not clearly communicated.

VIII. COMMUNICATION

Communication is a vital part of daily life and can be a conduit to lessening our problems. The focus of this chapter is on how we communicate and how often we take for granted the aspects of good communication.

Good communication means the bidirectionality of communication or, simply stated, being understood and understanding another. It's simplistic, yet both parts enable us to connect with another and this connection can occur either through shared experience or past experiences that bring us closer to each other.

You might have paid little mind to the previous statement, but it is of vital importance. Without direct communication, our physical, emotional, and mental needs go unfulfilled. Those needs are usually met through verbal channels as a more direct form, but nonverbal communication is also involved.

We have all been with a person who says one thing, but their body language suggests something else. For example, someone says that they are very excited to be involved in a project, but their body is turned to the side and you feel as though they are not present. Or, if you give a gift to someone and they say its great and thank you, but grimace as if saying "what am I going to be using this for."

How does communication tie into mental health? That's really a great question, and one for which I have a great answer. Typically, miscommunication can exacerbate our symptoms to include depression, anxiety, or whatever other psychological symptom one has. Miscommunication can also intensify the feeling one has of being alone, and being alone can lead to social withdrawal or isolation—all depressive symptoms.

We all seek to make some type of connection. Even a loner would like to be understood and be able to relate to someone. The only real way we can do this is to communicate or be with someone who has gone through similar experiences. Of course trained empathic professionals can also empathize and try to understand another's suffering, but having a connection with someone is usually a sought after goal.

Getting back to isolation, this can be one of the major symptoms of mental illness. If we look at the genesis of isolatory behavior, it seems to have its origins in miscommunication, which ultimately leads one to feel misunderstood. Think about it. Remember the times you felt the happiest, it was with people who understood you. That's when you felt the most connected.

One of the global truths is that we all seek people who can understand us. Think way back to the beginning of school, when you had to approach a new situation and you felt scared, shy, and anxious. If you were fortunate enough to meet another student who felt the same way, you both made a connection and your apprehensive feelings were decreased and in some ways soothed. You were "not alone" and could communicate to another how you were feeling as this connection strengthened and you shared in working through the feelings and experience.

Or, how about if you are in an elevator with another person and the elevator gets stuck. This trapped situation can produce multiple feelings, but with another person, the odds are you will come out of the situation in better spirits because you have someone to share the experience with. For instance, this other

71

person could be very positive, perhaps having survived numerous "locked in the elevator" situations or they could even be a fireman who is used to stressful situations like being stuck in enclosed spaces. These experienced people will be beneficial and you can take your social cues from them. Together, as you communicate your thoughts and feelings, your negative feelings might lessen as you both try to figure out a solution to the situation or, better yet, just cope until freed. This situation highlights active versus passive methods as well as making the most out of a situation and learning from others.

Suppose the person you are trapped with in the elevator has claustrophobia and begins to panic. Further, you learn that her father died in an elevator and she was once locked in her basement for days. This more difficult scenario is painted because, from these factors, one would expect that she will make "your stay with her" much more difficult and trying. Unless you're a very calm person trained to help this person, reworking her past negative experiences at the current time will be difficult.[3]

We each have differing viewpoints, usually based upon our own experience, and while one person may see a crisis during this situation, another may see an opportunity for a positive interaction or experience. The main point is that communication is vital to develop a connection and feel understood, while also highlighting how one's approach to a life situation or stressor can affect outcome.

In the elevator scenario with the firefighter, you can learn ways to stay calm from this man, while at the same time having the opportunity to talk to someone with a very different and interesting job. Asking a person if they have ever saved some-

---

[3] Reworking negative experiences into positive experiences typically involves psychotherapy and a more controlled and structured environment.

one or been in a life threatening situation and getting a positive reply would help ease the situation. Or better yet, how about finding out what made them get into the field they are in? All of these questions and the ability to communicate will allow you to 1) cope during the current situation, and 2) gain a connection or at least a way to understand someone with a different background.

As I write about this example, I am reminded of the Doritos commercial that showed four or five people stuck in an elevator after they had gone food shopping. Instead of panicking, they sit down, open up their groceries, and begin to enjoy each other's company while munching on their favorite snack Doritos. In this example, the focus is taken off the situation and re-centered onto food or the social situation. As they are enjoying the food and socialization, the elevator power comes back on, but one of the people in the elevator hits the emergency stop button so they can continue enjoying their time together.

Going through a stressful experience with another person has the potential to both strengthen your connection with another and build your relationship. Unfortunately, it can also create distance and alienate you among your peers. Let's look at a tragic example, the death of a child.

When a child dies, this is a very traumatic experience for both the parents and the community. In particular, parents struggle to cope with this loss. The problem typically centers on how each individual parent copes with loss, or more specifically with death and dying. One parent might isolate and pull away, whereas the other might want to talk about the loss and get supported and nurtured. As a couple, you might not be aware of your coping style during a time of tragedy because prior to this death, you never had to experience such a major setback or upsetting experience.

The outcome of such a devastating loss can either strengthen the existing relationship or it can rip it apart. Cognitively one might think "if we can get through this, we can get through anything," or "our marriage will not survive this tragedy."

In my clinical practice, during the initial loss of a child, parents are given this template and the explanation that each parent needs to respect the other's way of coping with death. I also highlight the process of working through a loss and point out the necessary factors and predictable responses. When one outlines the terrain or predicts the path ahead, it becomes easier for a person to travel that path. Although difficult, people prefer a predictable road so they can prepare themselves for the journey.

If, during this difficult time, the couple was able to communicate and get their needs of caring, nurturing, physical comfort, support...etc. met, then their connection grows and their relationship strengthens. If it goes the other way, each person will feel more alone, more isolated, and their despair will be more unique until they begin to realize how precious life is and their limitations on time, and that their individual relationship needs are not being met.

In other words, life is too short to feel so alone and empty, especially when you are with someone you "love." With an experience such as death, this sometimes can reinforce the realization that you never know how much time you have remaining. This realization crept up on society after the 9/11 attacks on the U.S. and specifically in New York City. What transpired after the events of 9/11 was that relationships either solidified or ended. Couples who had been dating for many years chose to get married. Other long-term couples ended their relationship and went their separate ways because they realized they did not want to waste anymore of their time with someone not in their future.

What people found out after such a life altering event was that life is short and that they needed to make the most of the time they had. Almost parodying the classic Crosby, Stills, Nash and Young song "Love the One you're With," couples decided to either grow together or separate. People soon realized that they were not going to waste anymore of their precious time.

These tales fit within this chapter because communication is vital and therefore extremely important. The main lesson is we all need to learn how to communicate our needs and desires. Prior to these tragedies, couples might not have focused so much on their communication and miscommunication probably ensued.

Fortunately, these folks were able to identify the difficulties in their relationships and make a drastic life change. Others might not have changed, but folks largely did get the inherent message that "life is very short" and it's important to live life to the fullest. In this way, they either maintained and improved happiness, or ended the relationship to seek out what they were looking for.

What makes communication so important? From my viewpoint, I hypothesize that "*if our needs are being met, we will not look elsewhere to meet them.*" In order to meet one's needs, we have to communicate such needs. If you communicate your needs to someone and they go unmet, then you have to make a choice about your relationship with this person. In other words, you now have the data about the unspoken question of whether an individual is responsive to you and your needs, assuming they are realistic.

The hypothesis sounds relatively simple, but applying it to life isn't easy, especially when communication between the sexes can be complicated. John Gray's bestselling book *Men are from Mars, and Woman are from Venus* highlighted the differences between men and women and focused on communication difficulties.

Remember, it is up to the individual to determine how to communicate and do so effectively. The ABC model provides the tools to change your life and live a more psychologically healthy life. Communication is just one more aspect involved in improving your life.

The importance of communication also extends to its opposite, that of miscommunication. If we miscommunicate, this goes against developing a connection and worsens misunderstanding. We also begin to feel alone and this isolatory feeling can lead to deteriorating mental health.

Again, we seek a connection with others and my hypothesis focuses on making a connection through learning and practicing how to communicate. This includes being able to communicate our wishes, desires, and needs. If this can be done and another person can understand us and meet our needs, there is a greater chance that you will feel healthy, connected, and satisfied. In addition, if miscommunication occurs, either party can correct the miscommunication and ensuing problems.

The feeling of connecting with another, that someone understands you and that you are not alone is paramount to a mentally healthy existence. We are social beings and studies have shown that happily married couples live longer and enjoy life more fully. Not wanting to get into a full-blown debate on the importance of marriage and relationships, I will just say that from time immemorial, growing up with others was vital to our survival (remember tribes with hunters and gatherers). Therefore, for your own personal wellbeing, I suggest working on ways to improve your communication, which can create better relationships. This includes direct communication, like saying what you mean and what you want, putting yourself in the other person's shoes (empathy), listening carefully to what they say, and even repeating to the other person what you heard so they know you understand them (a technique called parroting).

As I trained to become a psychologist, I learned how to listen through various methods. Specifically, I learned about reflecting people's statements, paraphrasing what they said, and really understanding them. I also learned to empathize with them and to really identify with how they feel. The reasons for this are quite simple. In order to help people make changes, you need to understand them and their life, including the context in which they were raised. This includes validating their feelings, being supportive, and understanding how they evolved or turned out the way they did.

We all want recognition and approval as well as a connection and strive to better ourselves. However, we sometimes are thrown off by negative experiences. Regardless of background, by learning these simple "tricks" to communication and working towards improving your relationships, life can begin to improve as you improve your communication to everyone.

In addition, if you begin to apply the ABC's and make behavioral changes, focus on your structure, identify your negative thoughts, and stay away from extremes, you can change your life for the better. We all have the power within ourselves to change our lives in the direction we want it to take. It just takes insight and hard work, yet it is very possible.

The difficulty I consistently see in mental health patients is in how people cope with stressors. Sometimes one does not see the problems in their coping strategy and having a professional help you see the problems can sometime lead to positive change. Other times we need to be empowered while identifying the alternative coping skills we need to use. Regardless, we all need to be cognizant of appropriate versus inappropriate coping strategies, and the ongoing struggle to find a balance in our life.

IX. APPROPRIATE VS INAPPROPRIATE COPING

What are the differences between appropriate and inappropriate coping mechanisms? One possible definition is that inappropriate behavior might equate to the old adage of anything taken to the extremes can be dangerous. In other words, too much food, sex, money, or exercise can be unhealthy, just as too little of each can also be unhealthy. The key to effective coping is to find a balance or a middle ground. Appropriate would be suitable to the moment or situation and fosters adaptation to an experience or stress. It can be an effective way to interact with one's environment in order to obtain the desired (and healthy) response.

In terms of inappropriate coping, the troublesome areas usually include drugs and alcohol. Basically, if you are feeling depressed or irritated and go out and have enough drinks that get you out of control, this would represent an INAPPROPRIATE coping mechanism. As an example, let's say an individual does this a few times a week, then drives an automobile and gets arrested for drunk driving. The coping skill used at that moment to de-stress produced more stress.

Another example is working at a job that produces stress and after work you go out for a drink to relieve some of the stress and pressure of the day. Since this behavior is reinforcing, you continue to do it over and over again. What ends up happening is that you come home later and later (not to mention driving under the influence) and sure enough your time at home decreases. This produces the effect of not paying attention to things at home including your spouse, children and household responsibilities. Thus, your relationships with them will begin to suffer. In addition, you begin to have health related problems, including liver problems, metabolism issues, and sleep difficulties. By continuing a behavior initially thought appropriate and helpful, it begins to become inappropriate as it causes more problems in life.

An appropriate coping mechanism allows you to cope with your problems and does not produce more problems. It is usually safe and effective and can lead to a reduction of stress. In this previous case, the manner of coping was inappropriate because there were many negative consequences. The inclusion of negative, unwanted consequences is what differentiates the troublesome versus suitable strategies and is a key component of mental health diagnoses.[4]

What also must be taken into account is that any behavior, in moderation, typically does not produce problems. The main point is that *extremes* should be avoided. Let's say you begin going to the gym after work, and you get into a routine and find that exercise helps you de-stress. Exercise is a good thing and is important not only for your mind, but also for your heart and body. As you continue to work out, you get quite involved, to the point of going 5 times a week, and working out from 1 to 2 hours per session. Generally, this is seen as a healthy coping mechanism, but what happens if you don't give your body the proper rest it needs? You begin to lose weight, and at the beginning, this is very reinforcing. After a while (maybe a month), your body does not heal quickly enough because you do not give yourself the proper time to recover and you might

---

[4] As defined in the *DSM-IV* (*Diagnostic & Statistical Manual, IV edition*).

start experiencing pain. Not wanting pain, you begin taking pain relievers such as Motrin and your dosage is increased as you continue to work out 5 days a week.

The problem with this scenario is that you are masking your pain with an NSAID (nonsteroidal anti-inflammatory drug) and have not allowed your body to heal. If you continue to work out despite the pain, serious injury can occur. Injury can lead to many more problems including greater pain, time off from work, and decreased quality of life. All of these problems originated from an extreme form of an activity and, although initially started for all intents and purposes as a positive adaptive strategy, led to more difficulties.

Suppose your marriage is on the rocks, and you decide to go to the gym to get some stress out. As explained in the previous chapter, communicating with your spouse is a good option, but one that was not chosen. At the gym over the long term, you start to see results and you're reinforced to continue. Thus, you start feeling better about yourself and continue going to the gym. Before long, you begin to notice that females (or males) in the gym start to "eye" you and begin flirting with you. Having never received so much "positive" attention, you enjoy the flirtations, but one thing ultimately leads to another and infidelity ensues. When your spouse finds out, this BEHAVIOR is not accepted and divorce proceedings begin.

Problematically, divorces in general are very stressful, and through this chain of events which began as a means to relieve your stress or cope, you have now exacerbated your stress as you begin to seek a divorce lawyer, expend more money, and start dealing with the end of a marriage or relationship. Although this relationship fiasco probably happened because your needs were not being met in the relationship, one could posit that by failing to communicate to your spouse what your needs were, resolvable problems eventually played out in a predictable negative way.

While this might be an extreme example, it nevertheless can and does happen. It shows that extremes in behavior (with limited insight into what is "troubling" you) can lead to problems beyond your wildest dreams. It's very important to recognize problems, take inventory of them, and identify ways to change.

In the previous example, the person did recognize he was overstressed and sought to address his stress by going to the gym and working out. What he failed to recognize was the antecedent to his stress, which was his relationship problems and maybe even problems at work. Going to the gym daily will not help with your relationship or with your job, just as a psychological pill will not change your problems. In order to address the stressful areas in your life, you must first be aware of them and then take the proper steps to address them.

In discussing appropriate versus inappropriate coping, one needs to maintain a delicate balance in order not to turn a coping mechanism into an inappropriate behavior. If one uses a coping mechanism over and over and is limited in their choice of coping mechanisms, this could lead to problems. Having a variety of ways to deal with stress and cope is one of the safer avenues to take because you are never fully dependent on one technique or strategy. The previous examples cited choices of exercise or food, but other coping mechanisms also can fall into this trap.

Regardless of strategy chosen, it's important to monitor the use of a coping mechanism so that it is not overused, but rather that it is used in moderation. It is also important to have alternative coping mechanisms in place in case one fails or cannot be used. For example, if one has an alcoholic beverage to relieve anxiety on occasion, it might not be too harmful. But what if the anxiety remains? Do you still use alcohol as a way to cope? If this feeling continues to plague you, find out what is causing your anxiety and what can be done about it by utilizing alternative coping mechanisms.

If anxiety occurs in certain situations, you must determine the cause of this anxiety. Gain some insight into the behavioral precursors or antecedents. Review your structure. Perhaps you are consuming too much caffeine or not getting enough sleep, or maybe your job is simply anxiety provoking.

For instance, consider the stress experienced by an air traffic controller or in the Department of Homeland Security. One would imagine that these jobs are very stressful and therefore someone working in this position would be equipped with multiple ways to deal with stress or anxiety. These could include going to the gym, talking to a significant other or to a professional, practicing yoga or meditation, and relaxing during vacations or finding moments in the day to decompress.

If we can all readily identify expected stressors, we can also recognize and try to find numerous ways to cope. We all have readily available coping skills for the unexpected or unpredictable stressors in life, such as health problems, loss of job or relationship issues.

The importance of utilizing coping mechanisms is that you will have more "tricks in your bag" and thus be able to adapt to life's circumstances more quickly. Also, it is important to recognize when a coping mechanism is no longer effective (as in the gym example above).

Another important consideration is developmentally appropriate coping mechanisms. Let me explain. As a child, one might have used the coping mechanism of "sticks and stones may break my bones but names will never hurt me." Unfortunately, as an adult this might not work for you. Or how about yelling and screaming at people. While this might have gotten attention as a child, your days of throwing tantrums are long gone. Or growing up as a child being self-absorbed or self-centered might have worked well for you within a chaotic home environment where no one cared about your needs, but currently it does not serve you well to form and maintain relationships.

A good example about developmentally appropriate coping comes from my experience with Veterans. They were trained to not deal with their feelings in the military. This training served them well, especially on the battlefield when a friend of yours gets wounded or shot and is bleeding. The solider might feel scared, angry, hurt, vulnerable, alone, or upset and while these might be valid feelings, if he was to focus on these feelings without any action, he might also get wounded or killed. You're trained to react and process later, and this served you well in order to ensure your survival.

Problematically, when you are not in a combat situation, this does not serve you well, especially when you have to interact with others and follow social cues. This is particularly evident in relationships or interactions as you are closed off to your feelings. In the work place, it can actually cause serious problems if you discount your co-workers feelings, or worse yet, your own feelings. Now sometimes returning Veterans are suffering more than just avoiding or denying feelings, and if this is the case, seek out professional help. There is a high percentage of returning soldiers now dealing with Post-traumatic Stress Disorder (PTSD) and one should seek counseling or therapy to be evaluated for this damaging illness.

Previously in the model defining chapters, we touched upon anger turned inward that Sigmund Freud called "depression." This is exactly what can happen when one previously coped with feelings by avoiding or denying them. In an entirely new and different situation, this coping mechanism is no longer effective. My point is that you need to take into account where you are developmentally in determining appropriate coping mechanisms and sometimes these need to be changed as you change (for better or for worse as you age and can no longer participate in physically strenuous activities, you will need another strategy).

Additionally, you need to take into account how effective or appropriate a technique is and determine if it is overused. If overused, determine how you can become dependent on such relief as alcohol, painkillers, or antianxiety drugs. You must consider what other options are available. Again, all of the factors discussed can lead to an outcome opposite of what you are seeking. Instead of improved psychological health, you might end up with dependent behaviors that lead to less freedom or control over your life and unintended negative consequences.

I have found that it is also vitally important to mention the use of **denial** as a coping mechanism in life and its alternative, which is to **embrace** the difficulty or problem. Many people with terrible past experiences feel pessimistic about their futures. Some might even feel hopeless and helpless and do not want to go on living. People who are feeling this way might cope by denying their experience. Unfortunately, while this denial has worked for you in the past, it doesn't mean it will work for you presently or in the future. If you are struggling with your life and the methods you previously used to cope are no longer working, you don't have to abandon your past ways of coping, but it might be time to try new ways and acquire new skills.

For instance, denying past experiences might prevent you from learning how to prevent similar problems in the future. It also invalidates your feelings. Reinforcing the denial of your feelings can lead to stunted development and interpersonal problems. Instead of relying on denial, try to **embrace** your past experience and the feelings associated with it.

If you've had horrific experiences and chose not to think about them or don't ever want to remember them, frankly I can't fault you for that. Perhaps working on accepting what happened to you, and even forgiving yourself or others in your life, is a way to gain control over the experience. It is preferable to the experience exerting control over you. This technique of **embracing** your painful past will allow you to move on and continue moving forward in your life because you work to achieve some closure with your past.

In addition, by learning how to do this for yourself, you will have gained the inner control of your past and recognized how it has constrained or controlled your life. This learned experience or inner strength could also be applied in future difficulties so that you build on this newfound inner strength. In this way, you have reframed your difficult past as a "learning experience" and are now able to cope with similar difficulties in a more effective way. Again, this is not to minimize or invalidate your feelings, but rather embrace and learn from them.

Further details about how you will make the change towards embracing rather than denying can be found in the Interventions Chapter. There I will identify the difference between coping versus processing and demonstrate how the latter can lead to lasting change. I mention it here to highlight this strategy or technique because it can be considered another way to cope appropriately or more effectively.

X. CORNERSTONE OF LIFE—
BALANCE AND FLEXIBILITY

The most important lesson in life that I have learned or continue to try and learn is maintaining BALANCE. Achieving a balance in all phases of life will make for a healthier, happier and potentially longer life. Exactly what is balance?

Balance is the ability to be centered or flexible in all situations, to not get overwhelmed or overheated during a discussion, encounter, or event in life. It is the ability to take the middle ground in a situation with both feet naturally planted on the ground. Visually, using the previously described continuum it looks like this:

```
A                    middle ground                    Z
0 -------------------------BALANCE-----------------------100
Black                    Grey                    White
```

where the goal is the *middle ground* or GREY or obtaining BALANCE. As an example, let's look at sports in terms of athletics and balance.

In baseball, in order to hit the ball properly, you need to shift your weight and be balanced. With throwing, you also need strong balance and proper follow through after the throw. Pitchers, when they pitch, are most effective when they follow through to a balanced position. In golf, a smooth flowing swing is produced by beginning and ending from a position of balance. In tennis, if your weight is balanced as you receive a serve, you have the ability to respond in any direction. It is the same thing with stealing a base in baseball, where one needs to be balanced.

Anytime you "lean" in a sport, you set yourself up for all sorts of problems because you are off balance. In boxing, balance is vital to throwing and taking punches. These examples all point out the importance of maintaining balance in sports. This also extends to life or a centering if you will. In order to be balanced, one needs to approach life with a flexible approach.

INFLEXIBLE

Let's start with an example of being inflexible. Assume you are driving to work and hit unusual traffic. Since you're not sure what is going on, you might wait it out to see if it clears. Typically, you drive to work on the same route, a routine behavior, and when a new situation arises, our means of coping or handling the situation is determined by our response.

As you sit in this traffic, you decide to find another route to work because you're not moving. If you're inflexible, you might continue to sit in the car, become more irritated and anxious, and your body will begin to show your frustration. Your blood pressure and heart rate might increase, gastric juices might begin to flow in your stomach, and tension might begin to mount in your neck, forming a knot. All this from traffic? Realistic? You bet.

However, if you preoccupy yourself with something else, you can cope with this stressor. Would this work? Some folks listen to their favorite music or get on their cell phone and begin catching up on telephone calls. Others might turn off the highway and get gasoline, go to the bathroom, or find a place to eat or get something to drink. It depends on how you cope and how flexible you are in using or trying different approaches.

Another more flexible individual might begin to map out alternate routes and think to himself, "Let me explore the city to find out other ways to get to work." In this case, flexibility has multiple rewards. It allows one to accomplish their goal of getting to their destination and, at the same time, relieve tension.

Cognitively, one might think "I can get out of this traffic, explore more parts of the city, and really get to know the area and maybe find new places I'd like to see in the city." Worst case, I am still moving and I am not feeling "stuck," which many people enjoy because they continue to just keep on moving.

If one were inflexible, they begin to say, "I am going to be late" or "this always happens" or "these dumb people, they can't drive" or "I hate this commute and my job and why am I always stuck in this traffic?" All these statements increase your anxiety and frustration. In a way, this might be the way one individual typically responds to situations, with a negative outlook. Perhaps they are simply in a bad mood and this is an atypical response, but generally, or behaviorally, people have a typical response style.

While repeating similar negative statements, you might also begin to clench your fist, bang on your car, or shout expletives. These behaviors and thoughts might begin to change your mood. Feelings of irritation and annoyance might increase and who knows how that will affect your next interaction with other people you see that day.

Physically, your increase in blood pressure, tight fisted hands and banging on the car could have an adverse impact.

Hypothetically, if you have hypertension and cholesterol problems, or perhaps a family history of stroke, heart attacks, or brain aneurisms, who knows what else might happen. My point is that by taking an angry approach, *instead of meeting the demands of the situation* with a more flexible approach, you can hurt yourself in a very real and physical way.

Another, more complicated example involves other people. This example is an interpersonal one where an individual at work does not do what they are supposed to do. This is going to get complicated, as it based upon multiple factors. The individual, called Joe Fog, did not complete an assignment at work that his team needs to complete. As a member of the team, you rightly get annoyed and feel angry. In addition, the evaluation and future compensation of the entire team depends on this project that now seems incomplete.

If you're a member of this team and you have a strong work ethic coupled with financial obligations at home, you might approach Joe Fog, confront him, and if Joe is unable to complete his assignment, take over and finish it for him. This of course solves the dilemma in the short term, but does not address the bigger problem of Joe's supposed inability to 1) complete the assignment, and 2) work as a team player. It also highlights your ability to be flexible, although it also shows you can be taken advantage of.

Let's look at all of the potential reactions and ways to interpret people's behavior. Your initial reaction was annoyance and anger followed by action because you did not want to let the team down. In fact, you might think Joe is either incompetent or dumb as a fox. In a way, Joe just might not like to do work, and by avoiding the completion date, he enables another person to take control and finish it. The result to him is doing less work, which might be his goal in the first place. Ever meet people like that? They probably failed to learn a work ethic at an early age, and one could hypothesize that either their mother or father were overzealous and always jumped in to finish a project or complete an assignment, or that there were no consequences for incomplete work. These folks probably learned to skate by at an early age and allow others to bail them out. Regardless of Joe's history, you and other co-workers feel like he is a lazy, smooth criminal.

How does something like this happen and why isn't anything done about it? My first thought is if the project is completed thanks to you bailing Joe out, other people might not recognize the fact that you were the "savior." Typically, people don't really want to know, and if Joe has been working at the company for a long time and is a "likeable" person, people might assume he does his job and is competent.

Problematically, if you get no appreciation from Joe or your teammates, you might begin to feel resentment that can affect future interactions and relationships. Others might identify what you did, but not give you recognition while readily identifying Joe as a schemer or one who gets over on people. Regardless of the specific individual feelings, ill feelings will begin to circulate at the office.

Although you met this team problem with a flexible response, your response now has created a history with this individual that was reinforcing to them. Behaviorally, you can choose another option that might give you the desired outcome, while not creating dependence. You can also cognitively think about choosing your battles, and by this I mean maybe helping out on this occasion but having a talk with Joe and the team leader to highlight this problem so that it does not happen again. By identifying options and exploring them, you can correct future difficulties.

In this example, you had taken a flexible approach and it might have served you well in the short term. Continuing to apply a flexible stance will always serve you best because it gives you many more options. But is being flexible being balanced?

While being flexible can be what I term "being in the grey" (for those black and white or dichotomous thinkers), being balanced is what I would term being at ease with yourself or finding an inner comfort. I think they are two separate notions and cannot be implemented separately. They are part and parcel. I think in order to be balanced one needs to be flexible, but the reverse is not true. You can be flexible or over-flexible and not be in balance. Take the example above; if this worker continues to bail out Joe Fog, she will be out of balance.

On the one hand, she will be accommodating to others and flexible in her choices, but in the end she will be out of balance because she will feel like her needs are not being met. I doubt she will have an inner peace or be at ease with herself. In this case, she might be flexible, but not balanced.

If this supposed woman has read this book, and used the ABC's and is self-aware of her coping skills, she would be able to identify when she is out of balance and work towards correcting this problem. Since she is flexible in her work situations, one might assume she can be flexible in other life situations. This flexibility will serve her well.

In addition, this woman has what Daniel Goleman calls "social intelligence" or the ability to understand the intricacies of social situations and really "read" people. She was able to read Joe Fog and hopefully implement a solution so that his behavior is not repetitive. If she were able to do this tactfully, without hurting the other person's feelings, then that would be a true testament to her social intelligence.

In summary, this chapter described a flexible approach and highlighted the importance of flexibility and balance. It showed how useful the ABC's are in achieving these goals. In the next chapters, the importance of individualizing your approach and coping are discussed. And in the last few chapters, the specific interventions and applications to achieve the desired change in your life using the ABC's are discussed.

XI. INDIVIDUALISM

The concept of individualism is very important to understand because what works for one person might not work for another. This book is not meant to be a recipe for success or a one-size fits all solution. What works for one individual might not necessarily work for you. Part of the challenge and difficulty in changing yourself is in identifying the things that work for you.

Individualism refers to individualizing your coping mechanisms or making them unique to you. As an example, some people cope well with structure and this includes going to the gym 2-3 times a week or going to temple or church two times a month. It also might include watching TV or movies, eating out, or being alone by the ocean. A central tenet of this is being able to find out how to self-soothe: to find different ways to relax and enjoy life. You need to be able to love yourself, and be able to treat yourself well so that you can relax and enjoy life. Being able to reward yourself is a staple of mental health.

Rewards can include long baths with candles, massages, watching your favorite movie or television show, preparing your favorite meal, eating your favorite meal, or socializing with good friends. It could mean talking on the phone, venting to others, writing in a journal, using your computer, or eating ice cream. The main point about individualism is that not all coping skills work for everyone and individuals need to find out what works best for them.

In the Behavior chapter, a variety of different activities were mentioned that could be used to cope. These activities are meant to give people options so that they can find the coping skills that work for them. Over time, try out different things and find out what works for you. Why is finding coping skills important and why is individualizing so important?

Americans typically value choice and freedom and people generally are very unique. Some people have certain likes and dislikes, and this is what makes us all special and unique. While variety can be the spice of life, it's important for each person to identify coping skills that work for them and to structure these into their daily life.

The skills incorporated in daily life WILL help you deal with the daily stressors in life. Individuals who have begun to accumulate various problems that led them to have difficulty coping with life forget to use the coping skills they had grown accustomed to using. They stopped implementing the structured activities in their lives that enabled them to cope with stress. Whether out of absence or neglect, their daily structured activities seemed to disappear one by one.

It is vital to recognize and try out different activities in the hopes of identifying the structure that works best for you as well as tailoring it to your daily life. These skills need to be individualized both to you and your daily life because as you get older, or as your life circumstances change, your needs change.

For example, in the past someone had predominantly used exercise as HIS coping strategy. He used to run many miles to relieve stress, and this was quite effective for him. His problem began when he started having knee problems, which happens frequently when you get older. He had trouble accepting his aging and the ensuing difficulties with his body. He exacerbated this problem by not coming up with another way to cope with stress, like one with less strain on his knees. He might have initially stopped the running and changed his physical activity to riding a recumbent bicycle. That would produce less strain on his knees because you do not have to support all your weight. Being creative and flexible in your thinking is a way to identify new solutions to problems and limit the difficulties of being "stuck" in one framework too.

He also might have tried new activities, from playing cards to intellectual coping techniques to spiritual pursuits. Whatever the technique, he needed to take a flexible and open approach and try new things that tailor the specific strategies to relieve his present stress. They have to be unique and individualized to your own personal preferences. It is important to remember that running on a bad knee will, in the long run, worsen your problems.

My point is that you are the most knowledgeable person about yourself and you have to apply this knowledge by CHOOSING what you will do in your life while taking into account the obstructions or limitations imposed. You know yourself best and know what activities will bring about the most satisfaction or reward. If you don't know, try different things and monitor your feelings after completing these activities. You can be the judge, and with data, you can be more accurate.

While this can be a daunting task or a challenge, if you embrace this challenge and accept it, you will not only feel but will actually have more control over your life. Because it is your life to live, I recommend identifying the best choice for you, taking into account your individual preferences and also making certain you are not hurting others. Of course, if you are "hurting" yourself, you may have to take a step back and first heal yourself. This pain or hurt can of course be physical, or more likely psychological in the form of depression or other destructive behaviors. If you notice an ongoing pattern of destructive behavior, and continue to repeat patterns that lead to problems in your life (social, work, health), it may be helpful to seek out professional help.

In other words, when you examine your individual tendencies and determine you are unhappy because of X, Y, or Z yet continue to maintain this behavior in a self-fulfilling prophecy type of way, it may be time to seek out a professional to tease out all that factors that continue to get in your way and prevent you from achieving your goals.

While admitting you have a problem is difficult at first, again, if you embrace your difficulties, you will find the greatest strength to tackle and change the problems. I highlight this difficulty because the ABC's are only one tool, and sometimes people need a more intensive repair. If we are to use a car analogy, sometimes all we need is an oil change, and with the right expertise and equipment, it is easy to get the job done and change the oil. Other times, a leak in your engine may lead to a more complicated problem that cannot be fixed by routine maintenance, and as such, professional help is indicated.

XII. APPLICATIONS TO DEPRESSION

Before reviewing interventions for depression, it would be helpful to define depression and examine its prevalence, and then discuss how the ABC model applies to the prevention of clinical depression.

Depression is one of the most common and treatable illnesses in the country. One in five women and one in ten men will develop it during their life. Depression is most common in lower socioeconomic groups and most likely to emerge in families with a positive history of depression. The National Institute of Mental Health (NIMH) estimates that 17.5 million individuals in the United States suffer from major depression or bipolar disorder and that this suffering costs society $30 billion annually.

Typical symptoms of depression include sad mood, feelings of hopelessness or helplessness, irritability, and change in sleep patterns, such as sleeping too much or too little. Other symptoms include feelings of worthlessness or excessive guilt, significant weight change (either loss or gain), anhedonia or loss of interest or pleasure in most activities, poor concentration, indecisiveness, discouragement, depressed mood most days, lack of energy, lethargy and recurrent thoughts of death or suicide.

To be diagnosed with a clinical depression, the symptoms have to *cause* significant distress or impairment in social, occupational, or other functional areas. Typically, having five or more of the symptoms listed above for more than two weeks signifies a clinical depression.

One major goal in addressing depressive symptoms is to intervene prior to the point of developing a clinical depression so one may avoid needing the professional help of a psychologist or psychiatrist. The best way to do this is to have an early intervention. In this way, an early intervention can prevent difficulties prior to them becoming a full-blown problem. The ABC model can effectively be used for prevention by identifying problems leading toward a clinical depression.

In order to identify the applications to prevention, please review the diagram below.

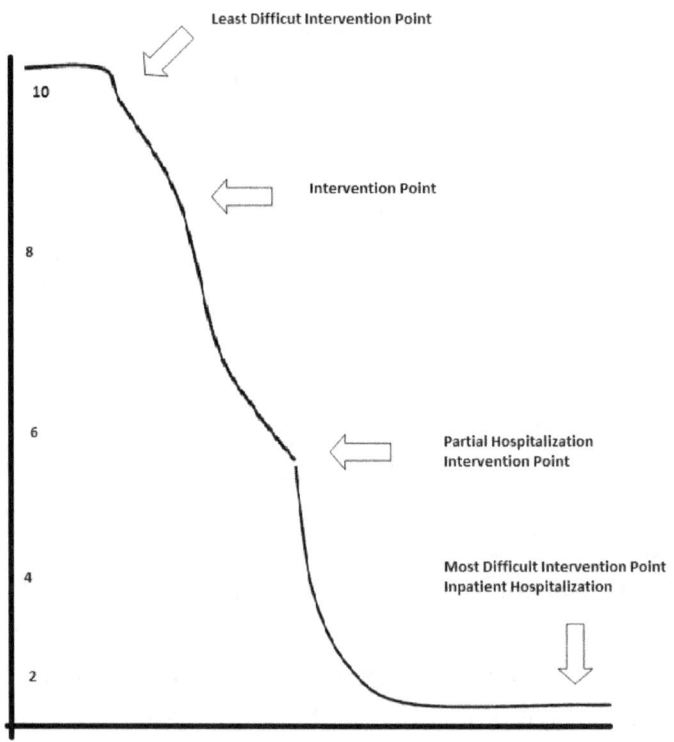

Basic Depression Path

As can be seen in the above diagram, the number 10 indicates the highest level of functioning while the number 0 indicates the lowest level. The diagram also indicates that intervention at an earlier point in time is easier than at a later point in time. This point cannot be stressed enough—as the old saying goes "an ounce of prevention is worth a pound of cure."

For instance, the more depressed a person becomes, the more resources and effort will be needed to get that person out of their depression. The diagram shows that the best place to intervene is when you begin to feel blue or a little sad. This could happen because of life events or other factors that begin to affect your daily functioning.

Application of the ABC's can include addressing structural changes, like not getting enough sleep or major changes in your schedule. This can include diet modifications, exercise changes, or health problems. It can also include relationship changes in terms of problems in a relationship, a recent break up of a relationship, or a brand new relationship that brings about positive yet new and sometimes challenging experiences.

In addition, recent life events can also bring about mood changes, like recent deaths or economic problems. Post 9/11, the world was an especially somber place. In New York, almost everyone was touched by someone who died and there was a creepy feeling of insecurity and depression in New York.

If you recently lost your job, economic circumstances can have a powerful influence on your mood, or if you started a new job or made a major life decision these events can weigh on you. In addition, the economy of the town you are in can also factor into your psyche or feelings, and the context of your life needs to be taken into account.

After paying attention to the structure of your life, and identifying any readily available changes, you might also want to begin to look at the ABC's of your life. If you begin to feel depressed after you leave your mother's house, or your girlfriend, and this feeling does not get better, you might want to look at how this behavior changes your mood and how it affects your thoughts.

Is preventing depression as easy as modifying some aspect of your life? The answer, of course, is it depends or yes and no. The model implies that you can identify the problems in your life, and by doing so, you can adjust them before they take hold and lead to lasting negative outcomes. The difficulty is first to identify the problems, and then change them.

If your cigarette smoking causes you to be winded when you exercise, and because of this you stop exercising, this might have a lasting impact. What if your exercise routine was the only way to reduce stress and maintain your health? What about that affair you're having; is that adding stress through the feeling of guilt? Or, what if you're in a dead end marriage where your needs are not being met? Will not addressing the problems make it change? What about communicating to your spouse to find out if you both recognize there are problems and if so, how to find natural and creative solutions that might be helpful.

The applications of the model indicate the ways to intervene, whether it be to a life crisis, feelings of anxiety, or increased depression. In a way, this model provides the tools to improve. One needs to use the tools in order to improve.

The key assumption for this model is that life events or behaviors cause us to have difficulties. The great strength about this assumption is that the solutions to our problems lie within it. This is because events can lead to difficulties and in a way you can control the outcomes by controlling the events to the best of your abilities. You can also control your response and determine a more effective or efficient way to handle problems by fully processing the ABC's. In a way, the model is built upon simple logic, with logical solutions coming from logical problems. The difficulty is that logic in our psychological life can sometimes be difficult to detect or interpret.

I find it amazing that we sometimes do not connect what happens in our life with our feelings or mental health. Many patients have said to me, "I didn't realize that was making me depressed, but it makes sense." It is like we have this built in haze when it comes to our psychological processes, but what I have found is that the more you practice recognizing and using the ABC's to guide you, the better you become at it.

I would also recommend taking comfort in the fact that psychology is still a very young science and we are only beginning to identify how our behavior shapes our thoughts and vice versa. Additionally, since we do not live in a bubble, other people's behavior also has a direct and powerful influence on our lives and also needs to be given proper weight. This means that our interactions with others can also cause many difficulties, and a dichotomous solution of saying "well, I just will be alone" may not provide the greatest solution.

Why do we lack insight into our psychic mind? The reason is that our brain protects us from either our impulses or primitive desires so we can control our behavior. If you believe in Freudian theory, our id drives us with basic instinctual urges and our superego tries to prevent attainment of these goals as it struggles to uphold a higher moral ground. Our thoughts are prevented from attaining consciousness to protect us and thereby allow us to more readily focus on the activities of daily life.

Because we lack insight, it is very important to recognize the impact of events in your life or your own behavior upon your mental state. <u>Recognition</u> is the first requirement in applying the ABC's. Although difficult, if you begin to think about your behavior prior to enacting it, and after completing it, and start to look at the impact it can have on other people, you will be begin to develop a greater self-understanding. This practiced skill can help you recognize various ways YOU contribute to your life difficulties.

The second step is <u>making a change</u> or intervention. Once you are aware of how your contributions affect you and other people, you can begin to change your behavior to improve your life. While not easy, it is vital that you stay with the change in behavior and maintain the required discipline to follow through with this change. The worst thing that can happen is that you quit or give up after implementing a change because it does not give you an immediate benefit or relief.

To assist with maintaining a hard life choice or change, I suggest applying the mantra "don't give yourself a choice when a choice does not exist." In other words, if you identify a harmful behavior, wipe that behavior from your repertoire. In this way, you no longer have that behavior as a choice and if you no longer deem it to be a choice, you will no longer do it (we all have a choice to jump from a tall building to feel the wind blow, but recognize the uncertain death is the result of such a choice, hence it does not become a choice). This extreme case shows that you can take away an option or choice for your own mental health.

Although change can be difficult, you wouldn't be reading this book if you were satisfied with your life. Typically, dissatisfaction can lead to making a change, and it takes discipline to implement and maintain a change. For instance, if staying in an unhealthy relationship maintains your depression, it will take inner strength to leave that unsatisfying relationship. While you might be scared of being alone and you might feel like you will "never find someone else (negative cognition)," being with this person is not making you happy.

Cognitively, you might think "at least I have someone" and "I will not find anyone better" while affectively you begin to feel depressed. Behaviorally, you stay with this person knowing that you are not happy. In fact, you might stay in an abusive relationship because of a history of witnessing or being involved in abuse, or because of the unknown and some negative self-esteem that motivates you to stay in the relationship because the next relationship could be worse! Your negative view of self and negative experiences needs to change in order for you to break out of this toxic relational pattern.

Whatever the reasons, you can either maintain your behavior and depression, or make a decision to change. Whether you seek professional help to break this pattern, or exercise discipline to break the abusive "chains of love," it will require a steadfastness and resolution to maintain change. In other words, you will have to be disciplined in your initial first step towards change and in not going back to "your old ways."

As is readily apparent from all of the many past examples, the utilization of all of the factors involved in the ABC model are important to apply to the prevention or amelioration of depression. Again, while not posed to be a simple solution to a complex, repeated problem, the ABC's provide the tools to

105

change if one chooses to incorporate change. It is with this guidance in mind that we come to some specific remedies for depression by using this broad based model, centered upon implementation.

XIII. INTERVENTIONS FOR DEPRESSION

This chapter discusses interventions and, more specifically, highlights a very important distinction when intervening against depression. The distinction comes from a difference in approaches for intervention. There are two basic approaches to reduce depression, either by COPING or by PROCESSING.

COPING, or dealing with the problem, is a very important skill to master. It involves identifying individual behaviors that work for you on a daily basis to help you deal with or manage stress. This can include physical exercise or working out, spirituality, or even basic tasks you enjoy every day.

When coping is discussed, it usually points to how you, as an individual, typically manage the stress you are under. Whether it is a cumulative effect or daily stress, we all need to identify ways to handle stress. This could also be writing about the problem, talking it out with friends, playing a stress relieving instrument or game, sports, exercise, or even crocheting. Whatever you implement, the techniques you use help to decrease your stress and allow you to continue carrying on.

PROCESSING, or understanding and working toward acceptance of a problem or loss, involves a more active approach where you are working to decrease the impact an event has over your life. This event could be a trauma, slight, or personal weakness. It is a process whereby you apply some mental energy to the struggle you are faced with and by doing this, lessen the hurt feelings you have and enable yourself to move ahead. These feelings can include anger, hurt, sadness, guilt, feeling mistreated, ashamed, or embarrassed.

Distinguishing these two types of method is important because while you need to use both to exist, only by the use of processing will you create lasting change. Let me elaborate on these approaches by using two other overarching concepts. The concepts I want to introduce are DENIAL and EMBRACE. These are useful for implementing change and understanding the differences between COPING and PROCESSING.

As we look at the diagram below, we begin to see the distinction between DENYING and EMBRACING.

DENIAL   VS   EMBRACE

Coping	Coping
Processing	Processing

Denial can be used as a coping mechanism, but it cannot be used to process past trauma. Embracing cannot be used to cope, but can be used to process past trauma to achieve lasting change. These differences are important with respect to ameliorating depression because one approach, DENIAL of problems, focuses on short term coping, while EMBRACING your problems focuses on processing these painful past experiences and making long-term changes.

As you think about the above distinctions, there are many ways to apply COPING or PROCESSING to your life. While these concepts are broad and have multiple applications, I will provide specific interventions below that can be easily implemented.

SPECIFIC INTERVENTIONS

On the following page is a simple chart you can generate called a Cognitive Behavioral Chart. This chart is easy to create and fill out, and by creating this chart, you can gather personal data about yourself. You can then use this data to make a change by identifying a ratio of behaviors that yields the most benefit. By working toward achieving the "ideal" ratio of behaviors that work for you in terms of the time you spend in each behavioral activity, you can improve your emotional wellbeing.

Specifically, this behavioral chart looks at our daily behaviors and you determine for yourself the amount of time needed in each set of activities to achieve the greatest satisfaction. It employs a basic self-monitoring technique to increase awareness and self-control, which can readily aid you in time management.

The method for carrying out this task is to increase self-awareness through self-monitoring. This is done through recording your daily activities for a specific period of time, typically a two week period. While this monitoring can be "annoying" in that one has to chart your behaviors and feelings, it enables you to gain awareness of how your time is being spent.

Created for this purpose is a chart that you can easily fill out. This is shown on the next page and helps you recognize your emerging behavioral patterns. The chart is divided into a time schedule and sectioned off by the hour and day of the week. It is comprised of the seven days of the week, and covers each daily twenty-four hour period.

Further, you can organize the labeling of the behavioral events into groupings of behavior. For instance, if you're in school, you can label your activities academics, play/social, sleep, and play/exercise.

WEEKLY BEHAVIORAL CHART

	Monday	Tuesday	Wednesday	Thursday	Friday	Saturday	Sunday
7am							
8am							
9am							
10am							
11am							
12pm							
1pm							
2pm							
3pm							
4pm							
5pm							
6pm							
7pm							
8pm							
9pm							
10pm							
11pm							
TOTAL							
P							
W							
S							

To make it easier to mark, I suggest creating a legend or guide. For instance, you could use A=Academics, Ps=Play/Social, Pwo=Play/Exercise, and S=Sleep. Or you could create a different legend depending on your daily activities and schedule. The four main self-ratings were derived initially by isolating our four distinct activities or behaviors. These are academics, play/social, and sleep. The play/social category was further divided into play/social and play/exercise to get better clarity on the various types of socialization. Although some people don't find exercise enjoyable and would not label it play, I have found it useful to place it in this category because it is something you are doing for yourself.

If you were interested in charting your meals for dieting purposes, you could add the category M-Meals. Sleep was really not of interest and was only recorded as a time marker for future comparisons. However, it can be used to determine how sleep affects mood or problems at work and is a major problem for a large percentage of the population.

For Sleep problems, I would try to get into a routine before bedtime, go to bed and wake up at the same time daily, and document the activities you do before you go to bed to make sure you have a good routine where your body associates the pre-bedtime activity (brushing teeth, washing dishes,...) with getting ready to go to bed. The research strongly equates routine with better sleep outcomes.

Getting back to the rating chart included in this chapter, we have three ratings of Academics, Play/Social, and Play/Exercise. These were the only ratings that were tabulated and depending on your issues or needs, you can create your own individualized rating scale.

Other ratings that can be recorded for students but not summarized to aid in time accountability purposes are: S=Sleep, C=Classes, Wa=Work Assistantship/Practicum/ Internship, Ac=Academic Class, Am=Academic Meeting, Ta=Teaching Assistantship, W=Work, Ex=Externship, X= Email time, and the headings of Breakfast, Lunch, and Dinner.

In order for this chart to be the most effective, it is suggested that you use 2-week intervals. The reason for 2-week intervals is that during the course of a week, you might not have a typical week or other events might interfere with what you would call "your normal week." By measuring over 2 week intervals, you can readily identify your behavioral patterns.

Further, after each successive week, it would be important to identify how you felt over the week so that you could attach to your measurements your feeling state. In this way, if you felt great after a week, you could identify the behavioral activities you participated in and how much of the time you spent in each activity. In this way, you are seeking to identify the best ratio of activities for you that lead to the most happiness.

By doing such charting, you gain valuable data about what works best for you each week. This is just one specific intervention where, through recognition of what time frame works best for you, you can learn to control the outcome of your feelings. In this way, you can implement activities into your weekly schedule that lead to happiness so that you achieve similar feelings. Remember, knowledge is power, and data is the king.

Observations from Baseline using this example.

A two week period was charted to ascertain a baseline for finding out approximately how much time was spent on academics and socialization. The results were found to be as follows:

Week 1: A=22.5hrs   Week 2: A=21hrs
Ps=9.5hrs   Ps=13.5hrs
Pw=1.5hrs   Pw=3.5hrs

While charting your daily life, you need to assess how you feel after a given time period, whether it is a week or two weeks. A simple statement such as I was happy, very happy, ecstatic or content can do or you can assign a number to it.

As an example, create a scale from 0 to 10, with zero feeling miserable, and 10 feeling ecstatic. By attaching a simple number to your cognitive behavioral chart, you can then determine if you are satisfied or need to make changes. If you solidify your schedule and implement changes, notice which change leads to the most happiness. Simply put, if you spend more of your time in activities you enjoy, you will be happier as measured by daily activities. This is not just a saying; it can be turned into a life plan with easy to achieve goals.

Many people have stated to me "I want to be happy" but when I ask them to clarify, to define what happiness means, they are unable to answer. This technique can help you define your happiness by delineating exactly what activities make you happy and the time you would like to spend in those activities on a daily basis.

By charting your time and overall feeling, you can replicate it on a daily basis. This will also give you power and choice; the ability to choose how you spend your time. Think I am kidding? Try it out, find out "what floats your boat" and arrange it so you spend more time doing this. Make it a life choice and you should become happier. It may take some creativity, limit setting, and sticking to your guns, but you can create a much better lifestyle by regulating how you spend your time. You can even reward yourself with more pleasant activities after completing difficult tasks. Think it through. The problem with this type of intervention is that you have to make choices and assume responsibility, rather than the status quo or just complaining about your lot in life. The use of this behavioral intervention is predicated on a simple theorem: *spend more time doing the things you like, and less time doing the things you dislike!*

Maybe some simple examples will help. You can either arrange your life to minimize activities that give you displeasure (i.e., being stuck in traffic—rearrange your schedule, work from home, take public transportation or create a way to have financial freedom so you don't have to commute) or you can arrange it around activities that give you pleasure. I know some folks out there will be jokesters and say "I want to be having sex all the time." Well, first off, have you ever tried this? I bet you will get bored and tire of this single activity. In addition, you probably need to find a partner to do this, and they may not want to do this activity all the time, and then reality will strike in that you have to earn a living.

Again, if this is what you want to do with all of your time, you may have found a new career to become a porn star in which most of your time would be spent having sex. I think this example illustrates my point that you can create the life you want by determining how you want to spend your time. If your activity schedule fails to give you the same pleasure, change it up again. The possibilities for your choices are end-less as is the feelings you obtain from your schedule.

Once you have your data, determine the best ratio for your individual life. Time eating, sleeping, working, paying bills, doing hobbies, exercising, family time…and try to model each week after your predetermined schedule. Work towards creating the strongest effect as you approach your desired ratio. The effects of meeting this ratio in my example were self-reported happiness and increased stability in daily life functioning (as a graduate student). I typically rated my feelings at the end of a week, like on a Friday evening or Sunday evening, because that felt like a good time to review either how difficult or how enjoyable it was.

With lifetime incidences of depression being reported as high as 18% (meaning that close to 1 in 5 people will experience depression during their lifetime), coming up with a plan to prevent depression, or put more positively, to have more enjoyment in life, seems like a great idea. This is but one way to address depression, but it can encompass your whole life. In addition, you may want to define all of the elements that give you happiness. Do you want to give back to others or society and volunteer? What about socializing? Do you want sodality, meaning being involved with a group for a specific purpose? Can you figure out or create a way to socialize (i.e., spend time with) people who make you happy? We have just added a complicating factor, but again it can lead to great happiness.

Let's say you do like to socialize with people from category X (college buddies, employees from X field, religious folks, folks of a certain political persuasion…), then how can you create a schedule where you are more involved with these groups or these quality people? Am I being to analytical?

Maybe, but the difference is that I am enabling you to create a roadmap and have choice, rather than sitting back and letting life pass you by without enjoying it or even knowing how you can enjoy it.

I can hear the objections now, "Dr. Goldberg, I am very shy, I am not sure I can do this." Well, my response is to start slow, build on your successes (basic behavioralism) by rewarding yourself so you can create/achieve the lifestyle you want. Life is not simple, but implementing the ABC's can simplify life choices and increase pleasurable activities.

If you really try to implement, gain control over your daily schedule, and have more fun yet still lack friends or a group, you may benefit from seeing a professional who can assist you in social skill building or processing your reservations. Psychologists, counselors, social workers, and even life coaches can help you to achieve this aspect of what is missing in your life.

If you have had a difficult life with a troubled upbringing and family, they can also help you process your past and gain acceptance of where you are currently and assist in guiding your future. Again, you are in the driver's seat and as scary as it sounds, you get to decide your future.

"Well, Dr. Goldberg, what if I screw up?" My simple answer, as any good psychologist would respond, is to reply with a question: "What would you do if you fell down?" Of course, the simple answer is dust yourself off and get back up, and the same thing applies if you make a mistake. Remember from the chapter on Communication, by having strong communication, if issues present in a relationship, you can work through the issues by communicating. Or at least determining where you stand in a relationship, if you are valued, how someone will treat you, and again, you have to make a choice if you want to be treated that way or devalued. Hard, difficult choices, but with a plan in hand and a belief in yourself as an agent of change, you can make hard choices that will have the best outcomes for you. While making changes can be difficult, they can be for the best, especially when you control what happens. Give it a try, even if it feels foreign!

XIV. OTHER APPLICATIONS

Other ways the ABC's can be applied include addressing anxiety. Many of my patients struggle with an over-anxious response to stimuli. While an initial response of anxiety can be helpful, there are other times when the response incapacitates you. Under the guidelines of the *DSM-IV* (*Diagnostic and Statistical Manual, 4th edition*), anxiety that is overwhelming can lead to social problems. When people experience too much anxiety and it translates into a clinical difficulty, this becomes a problem and typically requires professional help.

To address an anxious response, you need to identify your feelings (affect), sit with your feelings, and explore your alternatives. Let me explain what "SIT WITH YOUR FEELINGS MEANS."

Feelings are a good thing, although many of us choose not to acknowledge our feelings. When you have a feeling, allow it to register and try to "FEEL" it! This means there may very well be a reason for you to feel anxious, but if the feeling is debilitating (i.e., you can't leave the house for fear), then you need to gain control of this specific feeling during this specific circumstance. If you don't feel like you can gain control over this feeling, it will control you. This is the bottom line with anxiety, learning how to control IT rather than being controlled.

The research literature states that the best way to treat anxiety is from a combination of medications (anti-anxiety medications) and psychotherapy. Of course, either can work as well as learning coping skills for yourself. The ABC's can be applied so you can gain more control of your circumstances and reactions. In addition, with any type of anxiety, one's response is key. This includes social anxiety, PTSD (post-traumatic stress disorder), specific fears, and fears of leaving the house. Let me share an example of how to gain control.

Let us say you previously had an "incident" where you were scared. It could be a normal occurrence, where you were involved in a car accident or something bad happened in your life and you survived. Typically, one would expect an anxious response for a time, but after a certain amount of time has elapsed, one would expect you to resume your normal, daily life. I will use a personal example.

I was driving along the highway late at night visiting someone when a deer interrupted my path and trip. I was involved in an accident and my car, traveling at highway speeds, was no longer operable. I was ok, survived, but still was a little shaken. My plans had to be changed, I had to get a tow-truck, hotel, and call ahead to let the party that was expecting me know I would not be making it that night.

The traumatic response could begin after this incident because one could begin to associate "deer" (the agent involved in the accident) with danger. Matter of fact, this is exactly what happened. Since a friend of mine later picked me up but was too tired to drive, I was forced to get back behind the wheel, even though I was still shaken. In fact, I really did not want to drive but my friend had worked an overnight shift and was in no shape to drive because of being tired and fatigued. I was able to get a good night's sleep in the hotel, so being alert was not my problem. I was hyper-alert or vigilant with respect to being worried about another deer crossing my path.

By my friend unknowingly doing this, by me getting back into a vehicle the next morning and having to drive, I was able to conquer my potential fear. In other words, I was not given a choice because my friend was unable to drive. Because of this, with the accident still fresh in my mind, I had to cope with the past.

Now I will share that coping with a fresh accident that leads to increased anxiety is not easy. While driving back in the morning, I was hypervigilant, meaning I was on the lookout for the next deer that would cross my path. In fact, my driving was a little erratic in that I would get behind a car and follow them for a while because I thought there would be safety in numbers, yet after a while, if they were going too slow, I would pass and approach the next vehicle up ahead and repeat this behavior. Alas, this strategy, although not the safest or most efficient, kept me hyper-focused on the task at hand (driving) and led me to get to my destination safely.

Let us look into the ABC's of this example. My affect was fear/anxiety. My behavior was driving and changes in my driving behavior (speeding up to follow others) and my cognitions were "you are going to hit another deer." I even thought, "if I follow a car, there will be less chance of hitting a deer. In fact, maybe the car in front of me will hit the deer." In other words, I was justifying my behavior to reduce my anxiety since my behavior (driving) really couldn't change (needed to get to my destination).

By sitting with the experience (anxiety), and re-learning that driving does not lead to an accident (thankfully), I was able to re-condition myself and separate out an anxious response to a typically non-anxiety provoking behavior (driving). While it sounds easier that it is, one can master anxiety by using the ABC's and rehearsing the activity over and over again.

You can also teach yourself ways to relax while doing the anxiety provoking activity, like deep breathing, meditation, or other relaxation techniques so that you pair driving with relaxation rather than anxiety. If you can gain control and do this activity over and over, you will behaviorally reduce your anxiety and increase your confidence through multiple reinforcing successes. This is in fact what happened in this specific example, and after each time I drove, my hypervigilance and anxiety decreased.

The difficulty is "doing" the activity as most people want to avoid it (anxiety provoking events). The problem with avoiding driving (as was used in this example), for most of us, is that it is very difficult to get around without driving. Therefore, one needs to embrace the fear, use self-talk to change cognitions (I will be alright driving, I am scanning the area for animals, I have a cell phone in case something happens, it is daylight and there are less animals out,...) and maintain the behavior.

Again, it is very important to embrace change and want to change. Otherwise anxiety can incapacitate you. And while the ABC's can assist, sometimes one may need to seek professional help to address long standing patterns. The ABC's can help with preventing anxiety from getting out of control or incapacitating you if applied and used diligently but one has to want to change. Like the old psychotherapist joke: how many psychotherapists does it take to change a light bulb? One, but they have to want to change. The same applies to this model to address short or longstanding problems: one has to want to change.

XV. OBESITY

Obesity is the latest epidemic to become popular and one that can be difficult to control. If we look at obesity as a behavioral problem, meaning that we are not controlling the behavior of eating, then we can apply the ABC's to correct it. Another way to address obesity is covered in the next chapter on Mindfulness. This is an alternative cognitive-behavioral approach to reduce calorie consumption while being mindful of what you are putting in your mouth and also mindful of the eating experience. While the scope of this book will not get into the psychological reasons we overeat, we will cover ways to apply the ABC's to prevent or reduce overconsumption.

I do not want to oversimplify the problem of obesity, as it is complicated, but a simple energy equation helps to define the problem. WE gain weight when we take in more calories than we consume. In order to lose weight, you need to burn more calories than you take in, whether through speeding up your metabolism, burning more calories, or decreasing consumption.

While this is easy to define, it is much more difficult to lose weight without a lifestyle change. Let me repeat, you need a LIFESTYLE CHANGE! That could be as simple as giving up fattening, fried foods, desserts, high fat meats, or exercising a minimum of 45 minutes a day per the recommendation of the surgeon general. Now the latter recommendation I am sure will generate excuses and in reality, to be healthy, one should exercise this amount daily, but implementing this LIFESTYLE is quite another story. I would almost guarantee if you exercise over 45 minutes per day every day, you won't have a weight problem unless you eat while you exercise.

Even with exercise alone, that may not address the problem. One great suggestion is to document what you eat, and I mean document everything. Sometimes when we try to document, we tend not to document everything so that we do not have to admit to ourselves how much food (and calories) we are actually consuming. By embracing this strategy, you will see exactly how much you consume daily. Again, don't give yourself a choice when a choice does not exist. Document all the food you consume daily and in this way, you can determine your caloric intake using the data. From this, you can determine what specifically to reduce.

By documenting your food intake, some of the pleasure of food is removed because eating is associated with an administrative task as you chart your consumption. With data, we can make decisions similar to the behavioral charting introduced in the Interventions for Depression section that highlighted the use of a "weekly behavioral chart."

By documenting food intake and adding a calorie amount to each, you get a better idea of your full daily caloric intake. Even if you don't document calories, you can look at the consumption and point to the difficulties in losing weight. Most times, we are very surprised by how much food and drinks we consume and are shocked by the total caloric counts.

Psychologically speaking, if you are very overweight, major changes have to be implemented. The problem is if you derive great pleasure from eating, you need to replace that pleasure with something else, albeit more healthy. Exercise is a good topic, or a hobby like journaling, writing, or something else that you can do on your own and that gives you pleasure. Again, it is an individual choice but you must preplan this activity when you want to snack or eat junk so you have a readily available behavior you are able to implement.

You can also pair this behavioral change with a reward or goal. For instance, if you are trying to save money for clothes, a car, or another item, literally take the money you were going to spend on that latte, milkshake, burger, or other excessive food, and put it into an account for saving for that item. This will reinforce the behavior and combines to achieve both goals, losing weight and saving money for the item.

I would also reaffirm the statement "don't give a choice when a choice does not exist" as a mantra and guiding force. This means no excuses to "cheat." I have a rule, "no donuts." This does not mean on a rough day I can break the rule and have one. We all know psychologically that we will want to justify our behavior, and this rule takes away the potential to justify behavior. One must keep to it with no exceptions! The difficulty in changing our behavior is others who may want to pull us into our old routines.

As Nancy Reagan used to say, "just say no" and this needs to be reaffirmed. Don't give yourself a choice when a choice doesn't exist. If you want to lose weight, you have to give up things, period.

For example, if you create a 1,500 calorie a day limit, you can't willy-nilly choose when to employ it; it must be every day until you achieve your goal. By doing this, you will shrink your stomach, curb your appetite, feel good about yourself, and achieve your goals. There is no way that you will not lose weight when sticking to a limited caloric intake for a length of time. Of course, you should seek out medical care for monitoring of a serious calorie restricted diet, but without exception, the diet won't fail, we will! Don't give yourself a choice when a choice doesn't exist. If you make the decision to lose weight, it has to be a <u>fully committed choice</u>. This should also include an exercise program and a prevention plan.

A prevention plan is simply to have substitutes for typical behavior. Instead of potato chips each day, you have celery or carrots. Instead of chocolate, you have fresh fruit and monitor calories. You don't want to feel (Affect) like you are suffering, so you need to make it as realistic as possible to feel good about this daily menu. The best way to fail is not to set up alternatives or substitutes. The same goes for activities, like going out to dinner at a fancy restaurant with fattening food. Salads will be your best friend, with low calorie or no dressing. One needs to learn about appreciating the basics and in doing so, you will achieve your goals (cognitions).

It is also about feeling good, and by stepping outside of yourself when you crave junk food, you can reaffirm your behavior, leading to changes in affect and cognitions. One can say I am eating healthier to lose weight so that I can….(live a longer life, healthier life, meet someone to share my life with, fit into size…). You must reaffirm your behavior, otherwise you will quit. You must reward or reinforce your behavior, and no, I don't mean getting a caramel frappicino at Starbucks for 660 calories. Instead, maybe drink ice cold water with lemon, or a calorie free beverage with caffeine.

In any type of dieting, water is your friend. Drink tons of it, as it will fill you up. From the research, sometimes we mistake hunger for thirst and by knowing this, we can prevent that terrible, calorie consuming behavior by initially drinking water. Again, we are not dissecting the psychological reasons we eat certain types of food or overeat (feeling sad, mad, glad), but rather need to highlight that a food menu is not a punishment, that you are doing this behavior for the long term goal and good, and embrace this choice.

Now, if you have some masochist in you, and you need to cognitively state it is a punishment, and that will help you achieve your weight loss goal, you can implement the change using these cognitions. Typically it may not be the best approach, but as mentioned previously, an individualized intervention is the best solution.

Before closing this chapter, I will also add a strategy for eating out that may work. May I suggest asking for a doggie bag at the beginning of a meal and splitting your meal up into 2 portions, one which you pack away for the next day's lunch. By doing this, you avoid the possibility of overeating because the food is "out of sight and out of mind." This technique will save you calories and money in the long run. Another behavior technique you can use, if you are bold enough to implement, is to try and eat with your opposite hand. I can hear it now, "Dr. G, that is crazy." Crazy like a fox. Let me explain. By eating with the opposite hand, you are slowing down how quickly you consume food, which will then allow your stomach to catch up with your hands and enable your digestion to tell you when you are full. Since digestion takes 20-30 minutes, we usually consume too much food before registering that we are full. By changing hands, we are slowing it down. You can also work to chew your food 25 times each mouthful or have a slow, relaxing meal each time.

As I summarize this brief chapter, I would have to say you need to plan for potential problems, like wanting to eat junk food when something bad happens, and clearly delineate the alternative behavior for predicted problems. If you can plan out problem areas, and IMPLEMENT, you will achieve your goal. I would also make the plan very specific and tangible. With any behavioral intervention, you want to have tangible goals. I would suggest a diet or menu change for 4 weeks, measuring caloric intake each day, and having a set amount you can consume each day (1,500, 2,000, 2,500) and reaching it.

Weigh yourself weekly and list your beginning weight. Weight should go down each week, especially when you **consistently** stick to your plan. Set realistic goals, 2 lbs a week, 8 lbs for a month. When you achieve your goal, reward yourself with a nonfood item from the money you saved.

I would also determine your problem meal. For me, it is dinner, sitting on the couch watching TV because as we watch TV, we lose touch with how much we consume. We get lost in the entertainment and justify our behavior by stating cognitively something like this: "I worked hard and deserve to sit here, eat dinner, and relax."

Here is a radical intervention, get rid of your cable TV. Wow, Dr. Goldberg, that is extreme. Well, not really. Try walking, exercising, seeing new sites, museums, cultural experiences, or meeting new people instead. If you eat while watching TV, and you cut out the TV time, you are addressing a problem area. If I didn't watch TV while eating dinner, I would be more mindful of what I consume and it would prevent overeating.

I could also cut out dessert (don't give a choice when a choice doesn't exist). Don't buy it, and then I won't eat it! I know myself, and I am pretty lazy when it comes to going food shopping, so if I don't buy it when I food shop, I typically won't go back to the food store to buy the sweets. Now make sure you have a plan in place if you do finally get the urge for something sweet, make your own fruit smoothie or other appropriate alternative and monitor the calories you take in.

Imagine no TV, no desserts, healthier eating and lifestyle, and you need to find things to do with your added free time. You can go to the library (no eating allowed there), read a book you always wanted to (*War and Peace* anyone?), or write the novel or the article you always wanted to. Thinking/writing burns calories and is an activity, maybe even a reward. Or get back into activities you used to do, like gardening, walking, socializing (without food) and exercising.

In summary, create a solid, well thought out plan to cover your bases and areas of weakness. Identify your problem mealtime, problem foods, and emotional situations that can lead to emotional eating, and come up with alternatives. By planning out substitutes and alternatives to all the situations that arise, you will achieve your goal because you can implement your plan. Don't give yourself a choice when a choice does not exist. This cognitive reframe can help with the cheating we all try to do because it is human behavior. By validating our feelings and recognizing our limitations, we are able to address our problem areas/times and have a plan that can succeed.

Simply by monitoring calories and breaking it down by meal (breakfast, lunch, dinner), you can determine your "problem time." I met one mindful eater who had beans for lunch, just plain old beans. High in protein, it filled him up and allowed him to be productive without "wanting" other foods. It also was great on his wallet and if you rid yourself of cable TV (or TV), magically your bank account should climb. Maybe use the money for a new swimsuit, which in the past the thought of would send shivers down your back, but now you start to think, yeah, I could get into shape and look good. Maybe shop for smaller sized items to reinforce the changes. Again, you have to believe you can do it and that failure is not an option. Create a solid plan and stick to it—you will achieve it!

XVI. MINDFULNESS

Mindfulness is another useful mental health concept and is defined as being present "in your day in the moment." This is a very popular concept in mental health and I added this topic as it can be another useful skill to learn and apply for self-improvement.

For example, being mindful or present in your day to day life will give it more meaning. You will also be able to cut out behavior that is not intended, meaning activities you are not fully mindful of and that do not represent who you want to be.

There are so many times during the day that we are not mindful, like when stuck in traffic or during our morning routine of getting ready for work. There are other times, like watching TV or eating during meals, where not being present can lead to negative consequences, such as ongoing weight gain because one overeats or is not present to slowly enjoy each mouthful and therefore over consumes food.

The concept of mindfulness can also be applied to alcohol. If one is not mindful, they may consume too much alcohol, which can lead to negative consequences. Of course, if one has a goal of "getting drunk" then they really don't have to be mindful except that they are accomplishing their goal.

As a clinical psychologist, I may inquire into what purpose getting drunk serves, outside of forgetting life or avoiding a difficult topic. I would recommend embracing the issues as previously discussed and be present, but then again, I have seen many negative consequences result from alcohol consumption.

Getting back to the topic of mindful behavior, we all too often numb ourselves and therefore are not present. This chapter focuses on being in the moment and choosing your behavior carefully. In other words, apply the ABC's to the activity and determine what is leading your behavior. Is it thoughts (I want to get drunk so I can forget or avoid or not deal with x, y, z)? Is it emotions (I don't want to feel pain so I will numb myself, avoid, or "pretend" it doesn't exist)? I think if you use these negative coping strategies you will go through life in disguise, not fully appreciating your life and the control you have over it. This can be problematic but again it is a choice which would initially require insight. After insight, if one determines it is a problem, you can set about a way to change the problematic behavior using the ABC's or just the technique of being fully mindful in the activity.

We are all human beings with both faults and skills, and one need's to accept that within ourselves. If you don't like an aspect of your life or yourself, stand up for yourself and make a change. Be present and mindful in your day to day activities to either more fully appreciate each moment or the important moments or work to change the day to day activities you seek to avoid.

As an example, I got wrapped up in the day to day life when our pediatrician said to us, enjoy these days with your infant because they will go by very quickly. In this example, I have become especially mindful to pay attention to my son and really cherish the time we have together, especially since we are both getting older and for him, he is quickly developing. I do not want to look back and regret missing key moments in his life and not being able to be fully "present."

My suggestion for those who have new babies: marvel in the fascination he/she experiences learning new things. The same fascination can be applied to your day to day life. If your life is boring or you are avoiding life (and feelings), you may want to make a serious change, or if you feel it's too difficult, seek out some professional help.

As applied to daily life, try and be more mindful at work, during play, in your relationships, and in your life. Imagine working out and just trying to get to the end, rather than enjoy each moment. Life is a journey, not a destination and you need to enjoy the ride! The downside to having "wool over your eyes" in life or being absent minded (not focusing on each moment) is that life can pass you by. It can also lead to many negative consequences. Before you know it, you look back and have missed out on a good amount of time or a period in your life. Be present and experience the day to day moments that make our lives unique.

For example, being mindless can lead to car accidents when driving, overeating during meals, neglecting your job or relationship and undue stress without realizing you need to slow down and take some breaks. Ever taken a vacation and had clarity after it because you allowed yourself time to be, to think? Try implementing this strategy of giving yourself time to be in the moment more often.

I know many people who simply don't want time to think, analyze, or really take a life inventory of where they are or where they are going? It is kind of sad, not to plan out your destination out of avoidance or fear. Again, embrace and create the life you want by defining exactly what it is you want and making a plan with tangible goals to achieve it.

This type of old avoidance strategy comes from the "yes but-ers" where every solution is met with resistance. If you are unsatisfied in your life, you are not trapped in the same day to day drudgery, but rather chose to be stuck. Come up with a plan to get out of the repetition of a meaningless life and do it by making a plan to get out of it, one step at a time and follow through. This book should be empowering and can give you the skills to make simple changes first. In order to do this, one has to be open to life in the moment and obtain clarity and direction. Don't be afraid to live out your dream or make a career change.

Psychological studies have consistently pointed out that our most regretful memories are the times we did not try something rather than trying something and failing. If you try, you could be successful or if you fail, you can (read should) learn from your mistakes to improve your next decision or life change.

While I have heard it all, "Dr. Goldberg, you are a psychologist and playing with my mind," I am really not playing but rather shedding light on how we can get stuck in day to day ineffective patterns of life and how there are other opportunities and options out there. So, be mindful, in the moment, to see if you like your life. Determine if you are spending more time doing the things you want, and less time doing the things you dislike. If not, use the ABC's to make the necessary changes to improve satisfaction and happiness. And by being mindful, you will be more honest with yourself and be more truthful with your life and direction. The ABC's can help, and by empowering you to make changes and increase your hope for a better life, you can make the lasting changes you desire.

XVII. TRAUMATIC BRAIN INJURY

With the recent NFL season and wars in Iraq and Afghanistan, more attention has been brought to the suffering of a concussion or traumatic brain injury (TBI). A TBI is the result of a blow or jolt to the head or a penetrating head injury that disrupts the function of the brain. The severity of such an injury may range from "mild"—a brief change in mental status or consciousness—to "severe," an extended period of unconsciousness or amnesia after the injury.

The terms "concussion" and "mild TBI" (mTBI) are interchangeable. It is included in this book because it has taken on new significance related to sports injuries and injuries from the recent Wars. Together, there are about 1.2 million brain injuries a year in the USA from automobile accidents, sports, the military and general accidents. These accidents or injuries to the brain can have varying degrees of consequences, from temporary functional deficit to more permanent ones. The common theme on any of these injuries is what the best approach is to coping with the injury, and I have added this chapter because the ABC's readily apply to such life altering events.

From the recent Iraq and Afghanistan wars, this injury has increased as has its reporting. In the public, this is also a significant problem that can lead to short and long term deficits. In my work with the Defense and Veterans Brain Injury Center (DVBIC), we focused on diagnosing and treating brain injuries. Treatment can include working with neurologists for headaches, occupational and speech therapists for cognitive and speech related issues, psychologists to process losses, neuropsychologists to diagnose, nurses to manage the injury, social workers to counsel, support, and find referral sources, and various other health professionals. It can also be complicated by other injuries as is often the situation with wounded warriors. If you have broken bones, amputations, language issues or other ailments after or as a result from a TBI, one needs to address these difficulties as well.

If you have suffered a TBI, from a behavioral perspective, you may need to come up with other ways to adapt or cope. Usually with memory issues present in the majority of cases, the recommendation is to simplify your life and use various tools at your disposal like smartphones, calendars, simple mnemonics, routine, or structure.

If you are able to clearly think yet have other adaptation problems, applying the ABC's can help. If you are still cloudy post-injury, whether from painkillers or narcotics or the severity of the injury, you can obtain assistance to implement small, noticeable changes to improve your functioning and life.

From an affective light, sometimes brain injuries can lead to changes in feelings from the injury alone. You probably would benefit from seeking out a psychiatrist to address mood fluctuations or depression in a psychopharmacological direction. This really means if you are more depressed or anxious, start a trial of an antidepressant.

After a TBI, your brain chemistry may be off and implementing some pharmacological changes could be very important to your health. You may also have nightmares or difficulty processing a loss, for example if you had a car accident and you suffered a TBI while the other passenger involved died. This would be a serious issue in that you would have to process your grief and possibly associated guilt. Again, this is when simply applying the ABC's may not fully help and you would need to seek professional assistance (therapists).

In conclusion, this book and the application of the ABC Model are meant as a rubric or guide for our day to day navigation of life. As the subtitle of the book title implies, the Ten Chapters to Healing, by reviewing each of these ten primary chapters, one can use the strategies discussed and implement them to make positive changes in your life. By doing so, some of the mental health difficulties you may face can be addressed by exploring your individual affect, behavior and cognitions. Although this book is meant as a model and guide, in some specific instances, professional help is not only necessary but required.

For most of the examples cited and your own personal difficulties, you can use the ABC's to either change your thinking (cognitions), behavior, or mood (affect or feelings). The application of this model totally depends on you, but you can make small changes leading to positive outcomes and as you practice these specific tactics described from the ten primary chapters, you become better at applying this model. It is self-reinforcing.

My suggestion is to give the model a try, rate the changes and improvements, and if you are not satisfied, continue to explore the behavior, feelings and thoughts until you make the necessary changes to more fully enjoy the moments encompassing your days and life. It is through this continual feedback loop that you can improve your day to day life until you find the right balance using a flexible approach that incorporates spending more time doing the things you want, and spending less time doing the things you don't. Again, while this is a simple postulate, the old adage of practice makes perfect really is true and can lead to a more determined, stable, and enjoyable life.

REFERENCES

American Psychiatric Association. (1994). *Diagnostic and Statistical Manual of Mental Disorders* (4th ed.). APA: Washington, DC.

Goleman, Daniel. (1995). *Emotional Intelligence.* Bantam Book: New York, NY.

Keltner, Norman & Folks, David. *Psychotropic Drugs* (2nd ed.). C.V. Mosby: St. Louis, MO.

Kramer, Peter. (1997). *Listening To Prozac.* Penguin Group: New York, NY.

Redfield-Jamison, Kay. (1995). *An Unquiet Mind: A Memoir of Moods and Madness.* Vintage books: New York, NY.

www.ingramcontent.com/pod-product-compliance
Lightning Source LLC
Chambersburg PA
CBHW070141290526
45789CB00002B/581